Ergebnisse der Anatomie und Entwicklungsgeschichte
Advances in Anatomy, Embryology and Cell Biology
Revues d'anatomie et de morphologie expérimentale
Springer-Verlag Berlin Heidelberg New York

This journal publishes reviews and critical articles covering the entire field of normal anatomy (cytology, histology, cyto- and histochemistry, electron microscopy, macroscopy, experimental morphology and embryology and comparative anatomy). Papers dealing with anthropology and clinical morphology will also be accepted with the aim of encouraging co-operation between anatomy and related disciplines.

Papers, which may be in English, French or German, are normally commissioned, but original papers and communications may be submitted and will be considered so long as they deal with a subject comprehensively and meet the requirements of the Ergebnisse.

For speed of publication and breadth of distribution, this journal appears in single issues which can be purchased separately; 6 issues constitute one volume.

It is a fundamental condition that manuscripts submitted should not have been published elsewhere, in this or any other country, and the author must undertake not to publish elsewhere at a later date.

25 copies of each paper are supplied free of charge.

Les résultats publient des sommaires et des articles critiques concernant l'ensemble du domaine de l'anatomie normale (cytologie, histologie, cyto et histochimie, microscopie électronique, macroscopie, morphologie expérimentale, embryologie et anatomie comparée. Seront publiés en outre les articles traitant de l'anthropologie et de la morphologie clinique, en vue d'encourager la collaboration entre l'anatomie et les disciplines voisines.

Seront publiés en priorité les articles expressément demandés nous tiendrons toutefois compte des articles qui nous seront envoyés dans la mesure où ils traitent d'un sujet dans son ensemble et correspondent aux standards des «Résultats». Les publications seront faites en langues anglaise, allemande et française.

Dans l'intérêt d'une publication rapide et d'une large diffusion les travaux publiés paraitront dans des cahiers individuels, diffusés séparément: 6 cahiers forment un volume.

En principe, seuls les manuscrits qui n'ont encore été publiés ni dans le pays d'origine ni à l'étranger peuvent nous être soumis. L'auteur d'engage en outre à ne pas les publier ailleurs ultérieurement.

Les auteurs recevront 25 exemplaires gratuits de leur publication.

Die Ergebnisse dienen der Veröffentlichung zusammenfassender und kritischer Artikel aus dem Gesamtgebiet der normalen Anatomie (Cytologie, Histologie, Cyto- und Histochemie, Elektronenmikroskopie, Makroskopie, experimentelle Morphologie und Embryologie und vergleichende Anatomie). Aufgenommen werden ferner Arbeiten anthropologischen und morphologisch-klinischen Inhaltes, mit dem Ziel die Zusammenarbeit zwischen Anatomie und Nachbardisziplinen zu fördern.

Zur Veröffentlichung gelangen in erster Linie angeforderte Manuskripte, jedoch werden auch eingesandte Arbeiten und Originalmitteilungen berücksichtigt, sofern sie ein Gebiet umfassend abhandeln und den Anforderungen der „Ergebnisse" genügen. Die Veröffentlichungen erfolgen in englischer, deutscher oder französischer Sprache.

Die Arbeiten erscheinen im Interesse einer raschen Veröffentlichung und einer weiten Verbreitung als einzeln berechnete Hefte; je 6 Hefte bilden einen Band.

Grundsätzlich dürfen nur Manuskripte eingesandt werden, die vorher weder im Inland noch im Ausland veröffentlicht worden sind. Der Autor verpflichtet sich, sie auch nachträglich nicht an anderen Stellen zu publizieren.

Die Mitarbeiter erhalten von ihren Arbeiten zusammen 25 Freiexemplare.

Manuscripts should be addressed to/Envoyer les manuscrits à/Manuskripte sind zu senden an:

Prof. Dr. A. Brodal, Universitetet i Oslo, Anatomisk Institutt, Karl Johans Gate 47 (Domus Media), Oslo 1/Norwegen

Prof. W. Hild, Department of Anatomy, The University of Texas Medical Branch, Galveston, Texas 77550 (USA)

Prof. Dr. R. Ortmann, Anatomisches Institut der Universität, D-5000 Köln-Lindenthal, Lindenburg

Prof. Dr. T. H. Schiebler, Anatomisches Institut der Universität, Koellikerstraße 6, D-8700 Würzburg

Prof Dr. G. Töndury, Direktion der Anatomie, Gloriastraße 19, CH-8006 Zürich

Prof Dr. E. Wolff, Collège de France, Laboratoire d'Embryologie Expérimentale, 49 bis Avenue de la belle Gabrielle, Nogent-sur-Marne 49/France

Ergebnisse der Anatomie und Entwicklungsgeschichte
Advances in Anatomy, Embryology and Cell Biology
Revues d'anatomie et de morphologie expérimentale

46 · 4

Editors
A. Brodal, Oslo · W. Hild, Galveston · R. Ortmann, Köln
T. H. Schiebler, Würzburg · G. Töndury, Zürich · E. Wolff, Paris

E. Ramon-Moliner

Acetylthiocholinesterase Distribution in the Brain Stem of the Cat

With 18 Figures

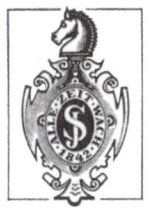

Springer-Verlag Berlin Heidelberg New York 1972

Dr. E. Ramon-Moliner
Department of Anatomy
Sherbrooke University, School of Medicine
Sherbrooke, Quebec, Canada

Supported by the Medical Research Council of Canada
Grant No. MA-1550

ISBN 978-3-540-06036-9   ISBN 978-3-642-50055-8 (eBook)
DOI 10.1007/978-3-642-50055-8

Contents

Introduction

The earliest studies on the regional distribution of acetylcholinesterase (AChE) within the central nervous system were based on the determination of the amount of CO_2 liberated by homogenates of selected areas in the presence of an ester of choline and a bicarbonate buffer. Using this biochemical approach, Burgen and Chipman (1951) were able to establish that acetylcholinesterase is not evenly distributed within the central nervous system. They found that the cerebellum, the lateral geniculate body, and the striatum contained a high concentration of AChE. The high concentration of AChE in the striatum could be correlated with a higher rate of acetylcholine synthesis. However, this was not the case for the cerebellum, where acetylcholine synthesis was very low. Other in vitro studies have been aimed at establishing the regional distribution of the other two components of the cholinergic system, cholinacetylase (ChA) and acetylcholine (ACh). An equally asymmetrical distribution for these substances has been established in vitro (MacIntosh, 1941; Feldberg and Mann, 1946; Feldberg and Vogt, 1948; MacIntosh and Oborin, 1953; Quastel, 1962; Mitchell, 1963; Krnjevic and Phillis, 1963; Aprison et al., 1964; McLennan, 1964; Cohen, 1956). The in vitro determination of acetylcholinesterase (Koelle, 1950; Burgen and Chipman, 1951; Giacobini, 1959; Bennett et al., 1966; Fahn and Côté, 1968; Miller et al., 1969) presents the advantage of permitting the use of a substrate like ACh which is a normally occurring ester of choline so that the establishment of enzyme specificity is less questionable. On the other hand, it does not lend itself to accurate histological localization. The detailed mapping of enzyme distribution became possible only with the advent of histochemical techniques for the demonstration of esterases. In Gomori's original technique (1948a, 1948b) esters of choline and long chained fatty acids were used as substrates. As a result, the technique lacked specificity and was soon abandoned. Koelle and Friedenwald (1949) introduced a technique based on the use of acetylthiocholine (AThCh) as a substrate. Since then, a number of variants of Koelle and Friedenwald's techniques have been proposed (Koelle, 1951; Shen et al., 1952; Pavin et al., 1953; Malmgren and Sylven, 1955; Bull et al., 1957; Holmstedt, 1957; Naik, 1963; Koelle and Gromadzki, 1966; Whittaker, 1969). Lewis' procedure (1961) appears to be one of the most successful modifications. In addition, other techniques have been elaborated for the precise localization at the electron microscopy level (Brown, 1961; Lewis and Shute, 1966; Shute and Lewis, 1966; Koelle et al., 1967; Lehrer and Ornstein, 1959). It should be emphasized that none of the above listed techniques uses as substrate the naturally occurring acetylcholine and that, as yet, only chemically related synthetic substances have been found to be useful for histochemical purposes, usually, acetylthiocholine (AThCh) and butyrylthiocholine (BuThCh). Strictly speaking, only the esterases of these substances, acetylthiocholinesterase (AThChE) and butyrylthiocholinesterase (BuThChE) have been demonstrated with histochemical methods.

The histochemical demonstration of cholinesterases has been extensively applied to the study of the nervous system and it is now generally accepted, in agreement with the earlier biochemical studies, that such esterases are far from being evenly distributed. Foldes *et al.* (1962) studied the distribution of AThChE and BuThChE in the human brain but, as yet, human material has not been the object of systematic investigation and, often, its study forms part of research carried out in a number of other animals (Bernsohn and Possley, 1957; Okinaka *et al.*, 1961; Friede, 1967; Papp, 1968). The same applies to the monkey brain. Friede (1966) studied the AThChE distribution within the brain stem of the spider monkey. The diencephalon and the basal ganglia of macacus rhesus have been studied by Oliver *et al.*, (1970a, 1970b). The monkey cerebellum has also been the object of investigation in a number of comparative studies (Friede and Fleming, 1964; Silver, 1967; Fahn and Côté, 1968; Shute and Lewis, 1969). The nervous tissue of the dog was studied by Hard and Peterson (1950), Gomori and Chessick (1953), and Abrahams *et al.*, (1957). General surveys of AChThE and BuThChE distribution in the rat brain have been carried out by Koelle (1952), Shute and Lewis (1963a, 1963b), Heading (1969). On the other hand, more or less cursory references to the distribution of these enzymes in the brain of this animal can be found in many investigations which are too numerous to be listed here (see: Gomori and Chessick, 1953; Brightman and Albers, 1959; Silver, 1967; Navaratnam and Lewis, 1970). The possibility of establishing phylogenetic trends in the appearance and the distribution of cholinesterases has encouraged many workers to study these enzymes from a comparative point of view. Gerebtzoff (1959) suggested that the older parts in the phylogeny of the brain would be the richest in cholinesterase. This hypothesis seems now less evident on the basis of the information gathered from a variety of animals: various ruminants (Bernsohn and Possley, 1957), the mouse (Siou, 1958), the sheep (Palmer and Ellerker, 1961), the rabbit (Papp and Bozsick, 1966), the red squirrel (Friede, 1966), the coypu (Girgis, 1967), the grivet monkey (Girgis, 1968), the miniature swine (Miller *et al.*, 1969) and the bush baby (Girgis, 1969). The non-mammalian brain has also been investigated: the frog (Shen *et al.*, 1955; Chacko and Cerf, 1960), the goldfish, box turtle and toad (Brightman and Albers, 1959), the iguana (Stolk, 1962). Perhaps the most comprehensive interpretative analysis of species differences according to cholinesterase distribution can be found in the work of Friede and Fleming (1964) and Friede (1966, 1967). There is evidence that the distribution of acetylcholinesterase in the adult brain differs from that of the developing brain. In other words, the maturation of the acetylcholinesterase system is attained at different ages according to the region or fibre system under study (Bonichon, 1961; Krnjevic and Silver, 1966; Endröczi *et al.*, 1967; Altman and Das, 1970).

A number of investigations deal with specific regions of the central nervous system. Of particular interest is the work carried out in the cerebellum (Friede and Fleming, 1964; Kasa *et al.*, 1965; Austin and Phillis, 1965; Bennett *et al.*, 1966; Silver, 1967; Altman and Das, 1970). It is remarkable that, in many species this region is supposedly rich in AChE, a fact that cannot be easily correlated with other biochemical and physiological findings, since the latter have often pointed to the possibility that cholinergic mechanisms in the cerebellum may be negligible or, at least, not nearly as important as in other regions of the brain (Curtis and Crawford, 1965; Crawford *et al.*, 1966). It is not possible to mention here all the work that is relevant to cholinergic systems of the cerebral cortex, although there are a number of papers that have dealt more extensively with this region (Pope, 1952; MacIntosh and Oborin, 1953; Okinaka et al., 1961; Mitchell, 1963; Krnjevic and Phillis, 1963; Krnjevic and Silver, 1963a, 1963b, 1965). An equally extensive literature deals with the AThChE content of the striatum. The reader is referred to the following relatively recent contributions: McLennan (1964) and Oliver et al. (1970a, 1970b). The cholinergic mechanisms in the lateral geniculate body, a structure which appears nearly always intensely stained in the material illustrated by many investigators, have also been studied by Curtis and Davis (1963) and by David et al. (1963). The cholinergic characteristics of the brain stem reticular formation have been analysed histochemically (Pavin, 1965; Papp and Bozsik, 1966) and, physiologically (Cordeau et al., 1963; George et al., 1964). The spinal cord constitutes another portion of the nervous system where histochemical studies (Roessman and Friede, 1966; Navaratnam and Lewis, 1970) can be confronted with physiological investigations, particularly the cholinergic system of the Renshaw cells (Eccles et al., 1954, 1956; Curtis and Eccles, 1958; Erulkar et al., 1968).

In addition to the above listed territories, which have been approached with histochemical as well as biological or physiological methods, several circumscribed areas of the brain have been investigated with Koelle and Friedenwald's technique or its variants: the hypoglossal nucleus and the dorsal vagal complex (Iijima et al., 1969; Lewis et al., 1970; Lewis and Flumerfelt, 1970), the area postrema (Iijima and Bourne, 1968), the area subpostrema (Gwyn and Wolstercroft, 1968), the various motoneuronal centers (Manolov, 1967), the cochlear nuclei (Osen and Roth, 1969), the superior colliculi (Siou, 1958; Hess, 1960), the thalamus (Olivier et al., 1970b), the hypothalamus (Abrahams et al., 1957; Peppler and Pearse, 1956; Hyyppä, 1969), the rhinencephalon (Girgis, 1967, 1968, 1969), the olfactory bulb (Sharma, 1968), the hippocampus, (Mathisen and Blackstad, 1964), the amygdala (Hall and GeneserJensen, 1971), and the salivatory center (Shute and Lewis, 1960).

Experimental lesions or interference with the normal function of the nervous system have proven to affect the enzyme distribution in various neural regions, nerves and fibre tracts (Sawyer, 1946; Hebb and Waites, 1956; Siou, 1958; Hess, 1960; Chacko and Cerf, 1960; Maletta and Timires, 1967). Of particular interest is the discovery made by Shute and Lewis (1961) that when an acetylcholinesterase-containing fibre tract is severed, the enzyme piles up in the proximal portion of the axon which is continuous with the perikaryon, while the distal portion becomes depleted. By means of this technique, a number of cholinergic pathways have been proposed within the central nervous system (Shute and Lewis, 1963a, 1963b, 1965, 1967, 1969; Lewis and Shute, 1967; Lewis et al., 1967).

The intracellular localization of the various components of the acetylcholine system has been studied by Hebb and Whittaker (1958), Fukuda and Koelle (1959), Giacobini (1959), and Whittaker and Sheridan (1965). In tissue cultures, Geiger and Stone (1962) have studied the localization of cholinesterase as well as the influence that various drugs have on this enzyme. The techniques for the ultrastructural localization of thiocholinesterases have gradually become improved and yielded surprisingly precise information on the distribution of these enzymes and their topographical relationships with the various cytoplasmic organelles (Lehrer and Ornstein, 1959; Brown, 1961; De Robertis et al., 1962; Barrnett, 1962;

Shute and Lewis, 1965; Lewis and Shute, 1965, 1969; Bloom and Barrnett, 1967; Erkänkö *et al.*, 1967; Koelle *et al.*, 1967).

The present work constitutes an attempt at mapping and parcellating the lower brain stem of the cat in terms of the degree of stainability of its various regions, when stained with Koelle and Friedenwald's technique for the demonstration of acetylthiocholinesterase (AThChE). It is concerned with the possible demarcation of territories which would be less evident with classical histological techniques and, to a lesser extent, with the assessment of the possible cholinergic character of the various areas and pathways. Special attention has been paid to the possibility of characterizing the reticular formation and finding out whether or not this vast territory deserves being studied as a single entity, i.e., as having histochemical properties which would justify a unitary notion in spite of its considerable extent. On the basis of the dendritic configuration prevailing in the various brain stem territories, an isodendritic core was postulated (Ramon-Moliner and Nauta, 1966; Ramon-Moliner, 1967, 1968) as a pool of possibly pluripotential neurons with long radiating dendrites which would form a continuum of overlapping dendritic fields within the brain stem. This core constitutes a matrix within which other nerve centers with more specialized dendritic patterns and, usually with more restricted connexions, appear enclosed. With certain restrictions, this isodendritic core corresponds to the territories usually regarded as reticular formation. Within this framework, the specificity of the AThChE technique was initially regarded as of secondary importance, so long as the technique would provide sufficient staining contrast for parcellation purposes.

The AThChE distribution in the brain stem of cat (Snell 1961; Friede, 1961, 1966, 1967; Abrahams, 1963; Holmes and Wolstencroft, 1964) is, in general, comparable to that found in the rat (Koelle, 1952) or the dog (Gomori and Chessick, 1953). The present systematic survey of the cat brain stem cannot be an exhaustive one since every region could by itself become the object of extensive study. Therefore, it is intended only as a panoramic preview of what further research may amplify.

Materials and Methods

Cats ranging in age between one and four months were sacrificed with nembutal. The brain stem was immediately removed and cut into slices about 1 cm thick following approximately the coronal planes recommended in standard atlases (Winkler and Potter, 1914; Snider and Niemer, 1961; Berman, 1968). The slices were immediately frozen and kept in the freezer at —10° C for a period lasting from 0 to 6 hours, awaiting the time for cryostat sectioning and staining. About 1 hour elcpsed between these two last procedures so that, while one set of sections was stained, a new one was obtained with the cryostat microtome. This allowed me to obtain a maximum of about 100 sections per day. Consequently, fourteen animals had to be sacrificed to obtain a complete series of sections, from the lower medulla oblongata to the caudal diencephalon. The sections obtained with the cryostat were allowed to dry on slides and, then, stained according to Gomori's (1952) description of Koelle and Friedenwald's technique (1949). For orientation purposes, other sets of sections from formalin-perfused animals were stained with cresylecht violet and with luxol fast blue. In addition, those sections which were immediately adjacent to the ones used for histochemistry, were stained with cresylecht violet. The incubation was carried out at room temperature at pH 6.4. In the present work, no histochemistry was carried out in formalin-fixed material and no control of the specificity of the reaction was performed by adding cholinesterase inhibitors to the incubation medium.

Observations

In AThChE stained material, the various territories of the cat brain stem differ from each other according to (a) the greater or lesser degree of stainability and (b) the sharpness with which they are outlined. The duality proposed by Mannen (1960) of "closed" nuclei versus "open" nuclei is as applicable here as in Golgi stained material. Some centers like the inferior olivary complex stand out not only because of their high enzyme content but also because of their strikingly well delimited borderlines. Others, like the superior olivary complex, are equally well delimited but remarkably pale. On the other hand, there are a number of regions, which may be either pale or intensely stained, that display very poorly delimited outlines so that the separation from adjacent areas becomes quite arbitrary. The following account is presented in terms of a working hodological classification of nerve centers. It should be borne in mind, however, that no striking correlations appear to exist between the functional role or hodological order of a given center and its AThChE content. Only general trends and rules subject to notorious exceptions can be suggested.

Motoneuronal Centers and Neighbor Regions

Koelle (1952) pointed out that the motoneuronal centers display a positive cholinesterase stain which could be due not only to the presence of "true" acetylcholinesterase but also to that of the non-specific cholinesterase(s). Manolov (1967) made a general survey of the cholinesterase content of the various motor nuclei of the brain stem of cat, rabbit, guinea pig and rat. In all animals, these centers are rich in AThChE and, in somes cases, also in BuThChE. In agreement with our observations, the rule whereby all motoneuronal centers are rich in enzyme appears to have no exceptions.

The staggering of the motor nuclei of the brain stem into two columns, branchiomeric and somatic, appears to suggest itself in AThChE material better than with other classical histological methods. It is difficult, for example, to determine the point where the n. ambiguus is replaced by the n. facialis. Similarly, the nuclei of the extrinsic eye muscles are linked by darkly stained regions which may not necessarily be populated by motor neurons but contribute, nevertheless, to the formation of an evident dorsal paramedian column within which the nuclei oculomotorius, trochlearis and abducens are embedded.

The *nucleus ambiguus* is very diffusely organized. Probably, the only legitimate way to identify this center should be on the basis of its retrograde degeneration following the section of the Xth nerve (See: Lewis *et al.*, 1970). Both in Nissl stained material and in Golgi material, it is difficult or impossible to differentiate its constituent neurons from those of the adjacent reticular formation. By contrast, in AThChE material it appears well delimited, particularly at the level of the rostral medulla (Fig. 8, in l). At more caudal levels, the center may be represented by scattered darkly stained spots (Fig. 7, in n and o). The nucleus ambiguus appears intensely stained in Snell's material (1961) where it can be seen as a relatively well delimited round dark structure, projecting forward into a lesser stained series of bands that extend as far as the most rostral portion of the nucleus of the lateral funiculus (or "reticularis" lateralis) of which they could form part (Fig. 8, in m).

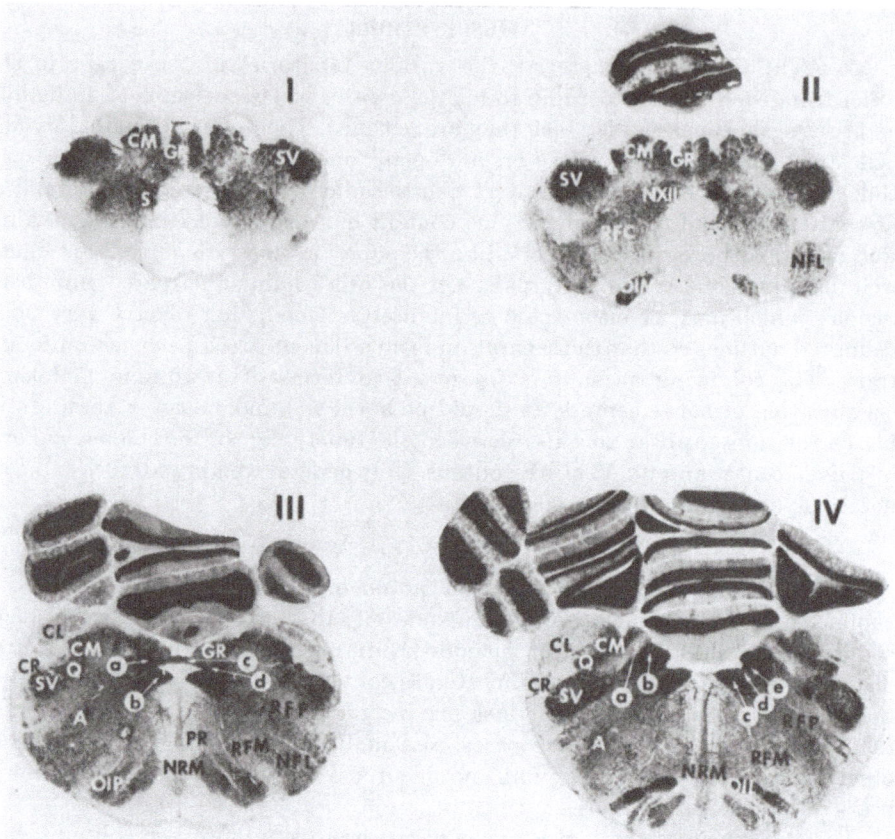

Fig. 1. AThChE stained sections of caudal brain stem of cat. The approximate corresponding stereotaxic planes are as follows: I—P 19; II—P 18; III—P 15; IV—P 12. In I, the nuclei gracilis (GR), cuneatus medialis (CM) spinalis trigeminii (SV) and supraspinatus (S) appear intensely stained, while the zona intermedia remains paler. In II, the nuclei hypoglossii (NXII) and olivaris inferior medialis (OIM) appear strongly stained. The nucleus funiculi lateralis (NFL) is also stained but not as intensely. The caudal reticular formation (RFC) shows only a weak stain. In III, one can appreciate the striking contrast between the strongly stained cuneatus medialis (CM) and the pale cuneatus lateralis (CL). The nucleus supratrigeminalis (Q) extends from the n. spinalis trigeminii (SV) to the latero-ventral portions of cuneatus medialis (CM). The nucleus ambiguus (A) appears slightly outlined against the pale background of the reticular formation although not as clearly as at more rostral levels. The inferior olivary complex (OIP) shows a positive reaction. However, not all its components show the same degree of stainability. The pararaphal nuclei (PR) are stained, although not very conspicuous as a result of being intercalated between fibre bundles. The nucleus raphe medullae oblongata (NRM) is poorly stained. Other regions relatively rich in enzyme: the lateral (a) and medial, or commissural, portion (c) of the n. tractus solitarius; and the nucleus hypoglossii (b). The latter are better demonstrated in Fig. 7. In IV, one observes, in addition to many features shown in III, the appearance of a pale band (a), medial to the n. cuneatus medialis (M), the nuclei of the hypoglossal nerve (c), intercalatus (d) and of dorsalis motorius of the vagus (e) are better delimited in Fig. 7

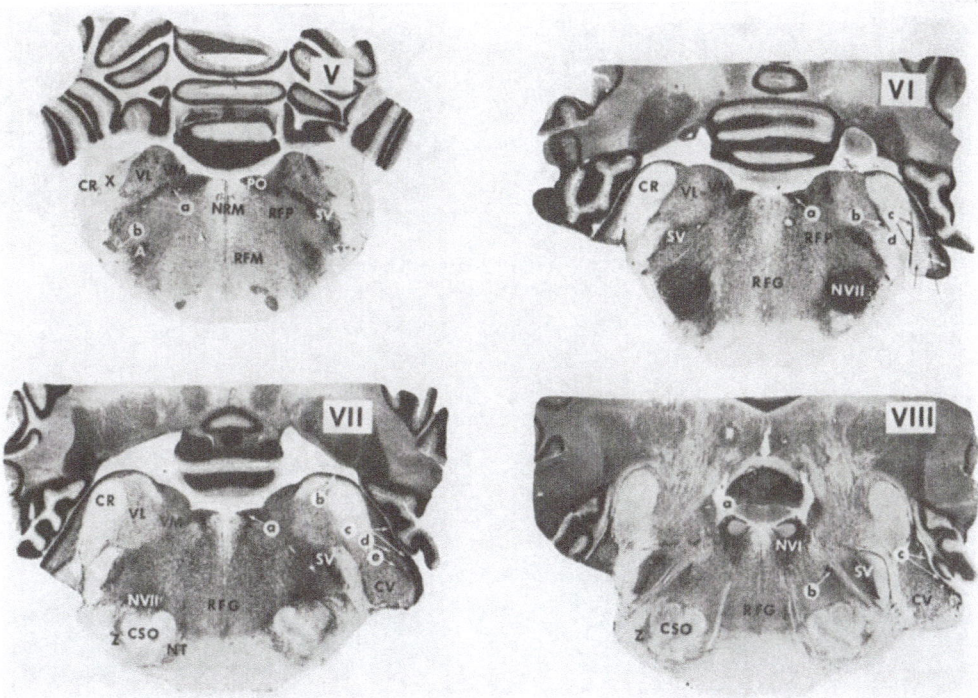

Fig. 2. AThChE stained sections of the rostral medulla oblongata and caudal pons. The approximate corresponding stereotaxic planes are: V—P10; VI—P9; VII—P8; VIII—P7. In V, the nuclei gracilis and cuneatus medialis, which were present at more caudal levels, have disappeared. They have been replaced by the vestibular "nuclei" lateralis (VL) and medialis (VM). Lateral to these, the most caudal portion of area X (X), lies in the region rostral to the nucleus cuneatus lateralis with which it can probably be equated. A positively stained band (a) bridges the n. spinalis trigeminii (SV) and the ventral portions of n. vestibularis medialis (VM). It may correspond to the nucleus supratrigeminalis (Q) visible in Fig. 1 III. The nucleus subtrigeminalis (b) is densely stained. It is not sure whether, at this level, the nucleus labeled A corresponds to the most rostral n. ambiguus or the most caudal n. facialis. In VI, the nucleus facialis (NVII) becomes very conspicuous as a result of the intensive positive reaction. The most superficial layers of the dorsal cochlear nucleus (d) are intensely stained, whereas the deeper layers of this nucleus and the ventral cochlar nucleus remain pale. A narrow, but very intensely stained band lies medial to the cochlear complex (c). In VII, the superior olivary complex (CSO) becomes striking as a result of its weak, nearly negative stain. As opposed to the facial nucleus, which lies caudal to this complex, it is considerably more pale than the adjacent tegmentum. The superficial layers of the dorsal cochlear nucleus (c), the striae acusticae (b) and certain interstitial cochlear regions (e) show strongly positive AChE stain. The deeper layers of the dorsal cochlear nucleus (d), and the ventral cochlear nucleus are weakly stained. A densely stained medial subventricular region (a) bridges the space between the n. prepositus hypoglossii (PO in Fig. 2 V) and the nucleus abducens (NVI in Fig. 2 VII). This region is described in the text as nucleus retroabducens. In VIII, the nucleus abducens (NVI) appears intensely stained, surrounding the genu of the facial nerve. Lateral to it (a), lies the relatively densely stained "nucleus" vestibularis superior. The nucleus spinalis trigemini (SV) remains darkly stained. Medial to it appears a dark area (b) which may correspond to the most caudal portion of the masticatory nucleus which becomes clearly outlined in Fig. 3 IX. The nucleus cochlearis ventralis (CV) remains relatively pale and is bordered by a thin, positively stained layer (c) which represents the most rostral continuation of the dorsal cochlear complex

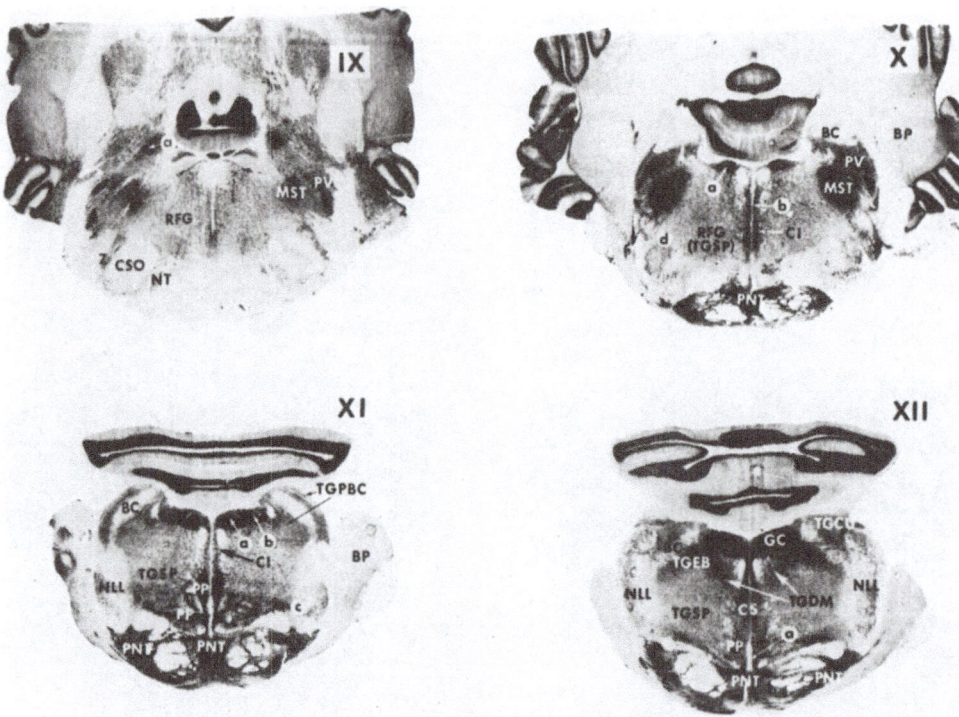

Fig. 3. AThChE stained transverse sections of pons of cat. The approximate corresponding stereotaxic planes are as follows: IX—P6.5; X—P5.5; XI—P4.5; XII—P3.5. In IX, appears the nucleus masticatorius (MST) intensely stained, medial to the nucleus principalis trigeminii (PV), also intensely stained. At this level, the "nucleus" giganto-cellularis (RFG) of the rostral reticular formation (tegmentum), is relatively pale. The raphe is also pale. No special features characterize the pararaphal region. In X, both the masticatory and the principal nucleus of the trigeminal nerve appear intensely stained. There is a subventricular area (a) which appears intensely stained, like the nucleus abducens, which lies caudal to it. In the text, this area is described as nucleus preabducens. At this level, the tegmentum suprapontinus (TGSP) retains the relatively weak stain that characterizes most of the caudal regions of the brain stem reticular formation. The raphe region, however, becomes occupied by an intensely stained paramedian region, the nucleus tegmentosus centralis inferior (CI). The pontine nuclei (PNT) appear intensely stained and some islands of positively stained material appear interposed between the bundles of the brachium pontis. In the text, this region is described as corpus pontocuneatus (d). In XI, the most caudal portion of the retroaqueductal gray matter appears intensely stained, with a lateral region (b) of diffuse characteristics and a round, relatively encapsulated center (a), the nucleus tegmentosus dorsalis of Gudden. In the paramedian region, a number of irregularly distributed cell masses, though often symmetrical, form the nucleus papilliformis (PP). The tegmentum suprapontinus (TGSP), the caudal peribrachial tegmentum (TGPBC) and the nucleus of the lateral lemniscus (NLL) show a relatively pale stain. The lateral extension of the pontine nuclei (c) appears to be continuous with the islands of the corpus pontocuneatus. In XII, the brachium conjunctivum (BC) separates a dorsal region, the tegmentum cuneiformis (TGCU) which is relatively pale, from a ventral region, the tegmentum entobrachialis (TGEB) which is more densely stained. In the midline, the nucleus centralis superior (CS) replaces, partially, the n. papillioformis. The latter is represented by islands embedded either in the tegmentum suprapontius (TGSP) or within the nucleus centralis superior. The latter appears stained, although not as dark as the n. papillioformis. In the midline a region rich in sagittal fibres (a) stands out as a non-stained structure

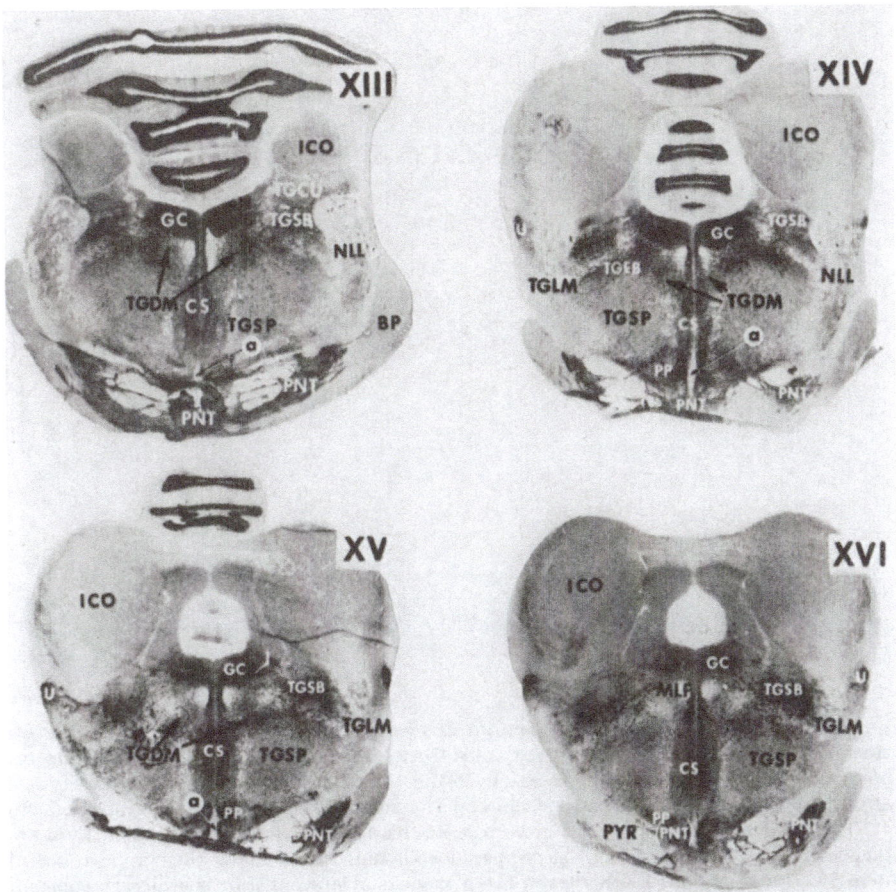

Fig. 4. AThChE stained transverse sections of rostral pons and caudal mesencephalon. The approximate corresponding stereotaxic planes are: XIII—P 2.5; XIV—P1.5; XV—P0.5; XVI—A 0.5. In XIII the peribrachial region is densely stained. As a result of the ventral displacement of the brachium conjunctivum, a portion of the darkly stained tegmentum lies now dorsal to it. This tegmentum suprabrachialis (TGSB) constitutes the rostral continuation of the tegmentum entobrachialis and becomes larger at rostral levels while the latter becomes smaller. It differs from the tegmentum cuneiformis (TGCU) in the fact that the latter is weakly stained. The nucleus tegmentosus centralis superior (CS) is well developed at this level. The inferior colliculus (ICO) and the nucleus of the lateral lemniscus (NLL) show very weak AThChE stain. In XIV, the brachium conjunctivum is still evident as a weakly stained area that separates the tegmentum entobrachialis (TGEB) from the tegmentum suprabrachialis (TGSB) The griseum centralis (GC), and these two tegmental areas, constitute a densely stained dorsal mesencephalic area which becomes continuous in its medial portion with the equally densely stained tegmentum dorsomedialis (TGDM). The nucleus tegmentosus profundus of Gudden constitutes a well outlined center embedded within this region. It is not illustrated, but can be found in sections lying between XIV und XV. The most important change observable in XV and XVI is the general decrease in the intensity of the AThChE stain in the peribrachial region and in the griseum centralis. The tegmentum suprabrachialis (TGSB) remains characterized by its relatively positive reaction

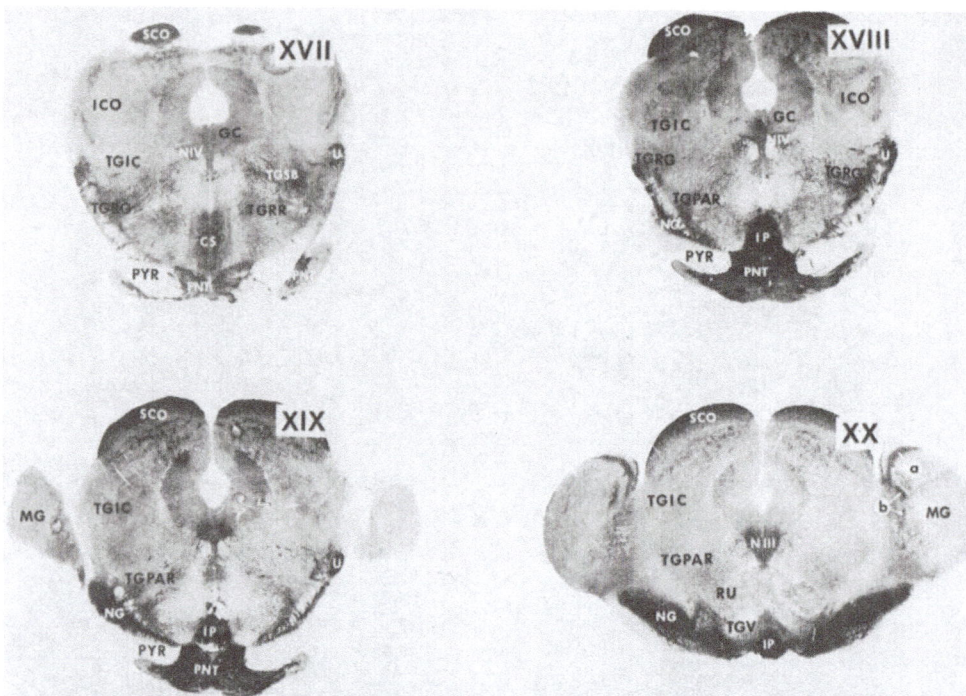

Fig. 5. AThChE stained transverse sections of mesencephalon. The approximate stereotaxic planes are: XVII—A1; XVIII—A2; XIX—A3; XX—A4. The right hand side of the photographs corresponds to a more caudal plane than the left hand side. The densely stained tegmentum suprabrachialis is still visible on the right (TGSB) but has disappeared on the left. The griseum centralis (GC) is more pale at this level of the mesencephalon than at any other level. The dorsal layers of the superior colliculus (SCO) make their appearance as an intensely stained region. At this level, the nucleus centralis superior is still very conspicuous (CS). Some densely stained strands, dorsolateral to the medial longitudinal fasciculus, indicate the most caudal extremity of nucleus trochlearis (NIV). In U, one sees an area which is well outlined at caudal levels, sometimes referred to as nucleus sagulum, and described in the text as the most caudal portion of the tegmentum retrogeniculatus (TGRG). In XVIII, the brachia conjunctiva decussate. On each side lies the mesencephalic tegmentum which, at this level, is relatively pale. It can be arbitrarily divided into a more dorsal area, or tegmentum infracollicularis (TGIC) and a more ventral one, or tegmentum pararubralis (TGPAR). The nucleus interpeduncularis (IP) appears as an extremely well delimited structure. The substantia nigra (NG) makes its appearance at this level, where it seems to be continuous with the tegmentum retrogeniculatum (TGRG). The superficial layers of the superior colliculus (SCO) appear densely stained. The nucleus trochlearis (NIV) appears relatively dark and the same applies to the median griseum centralis (GC). In XIX, on the left hand side, the substantia nigra (NG) is already well developed and shows an intense stain. The medial geniculate body makes its appearance as a relatively pale structure (MG). The ventromedian griseum centrale is darkly stained. In the superior colliculus (SCO), the superficial layers appear well stained in an homogeneous manner, whereas the deeper layers show a spotted or streaked appearance. In XX, the nucleus oculomotorius principalis (NIII) appears well delimited. The substantia nigra is massively stained (NG) whereas the red nucleus (RU) and the tegmentum infracollicularis (TGIC) and pararubralis (TGPAR) are very pale. The most caudal extension of the nucleus reticularis thalami (a) appears as a darkly stained sheath covering the dorsomedial pole of the medial geniculate body (MG). Medial to the latter lie some positively stained islands (b). Ventromedial to the medial geniculate body is a region, triangular in shape, the tegmentum paralemniscalis (TGPL) which is slightly darker than the tegmentum pararubralis (TGPAR)

The *nucleus facialis* (Fig. 2 VI, in NVII) appears as a densely stained round mass, immediately caudal to the superior olivary complex. It is lens-shaped, so that in sagittal sections its outline is not round but elongated due to the fact that its equator lies perpendicular to the main axis of the brain stem. In AThChE material its boundaries appear better outlined than in Nissl or Golgi material. In particular, it offers a striking contrast with the pale superior olivary complex. Owing to this contrast, the latter structure can be easily recognized at caudal levels where it has not yet attained its full extent (see pale region ventral to NVII in Fig. 2 VI). The facial nucleus appears intensely and evenly stained in its ventro-medial portion. Its laterodorsal portion is trabeculated and appears to extend more in a rostrocaudal direction than the ventromedial one. It is not possible to establish with certainty whether or not the most caudal strands belong to this center or to the nucleus ambiguus. The superior periolivary complex (Fig. 2 VII, in Z) extends caudally to form a moderately stained zone which envelopes the most ventral portion of the facial nucleus.

The *nucleus masticatorius* (MST in Figs. 3 IX and 3 X) is located at the dorso-lateral upper pons, medial and ventral to the principal sensory nucleus of the trigeminal nerve. Of all the motoneuronal centers of the brain stem, this one is populated by the largest neurons. It is shaped like a disc so that in sagittal sections it appears elongated, whereas in transverse sections it appears round. It extends from a plane immediately caudal to the tegmentum entobrachialis to a plane passing through the middle of the pons, at the level of the most rostral pole of the nucleus abducens. In transverse sections it attains its widest extent at the point where the superior cerebellar peduncle enters the brain stem (Figs. 3, 10). In AThChE stained sections it appears intensely stained and well outlined. A slightly lighter band separates this center from the principal trigeminal nucleus. Ventrally, the nucleus appears to be continued by certain strands of darkly stained material. However this region must be regarded as having an entirely different significance. It probably forms part of the corpus ponto-cuneatus (Fig. 3 X, in d). In Golgi material it is populated by allodendritic neurons somewhat similar to those of the pontine nuclei (Ramon-Moliner, 1968).

In AThChE sections a nearly uninterrupted paramedian dorsal column of more or less intensely stained regions extends from the most rostral portion of the mesencephalon to the level of the obex. Although the centers embedded in this column have very diverse functions and connexions, the trend deserves to be pointed out as it could reflect some common physiological property as yet un-determined. This column includes, in a caudorostral sequence, the area postrema, the nucleus hypoglossii, the dorsal complex of the vagus, the n. prepositus hypo-glossii, the n. retroabducens, the n. abducens, the n. preabducens, the ponto-mesencephalic central gray matter, the nucleus trochlearis, the nucleus oculomo-torius, the nuclei of Perlia and Edinger-Westphal, and a number of undenominated subventricular and periaqueductal regions.

In our AThChE material, the nucleus hypoglossii (NXII in Fig. 1 II) is in-tensely stained. However, it appears (Iijima *et al.*, 1969; Lewis and Flumerfelt, 1970) that this center is richer in BuThChE than in AThChE, a peculiarity that differentiates it from the adjacent dorsal motor nucleus of the vagus. The nucleus hypoglossii offers a very sharp medioventral boundary which separates it from the

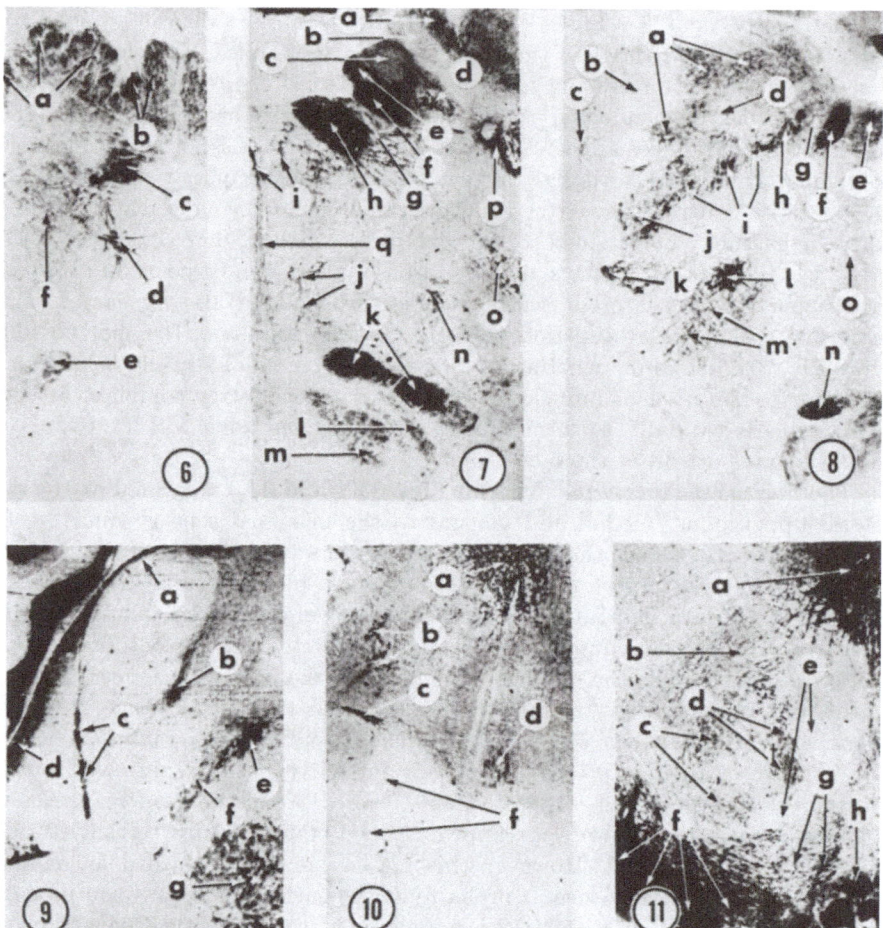

Fig. 6. Caudal medulla oblongata (approximately, stereotaxic plane P 15). Both the dorsal portion of the nucleus cuneatus medialis (a) and gracilis (b) display an irregular pattern with alternating dense and light areas. The hypoglossal nucleus (c) and the nucleus supraspinatus (d) are evenly and densely stained. The most caudal pole of the nucleus olivaris inferior medialis (e) is moderately stained. The zona intermedia or caudal reticular formation (f) remains pale

Fig. 7. Medulla oblongata (approximately, stereotaxic plane P 12). The fasciculus solitarius (d) lies lateral to its nucleus which is formed by a dark, peripheral ring and a lighter core (c). Medial to this complex, and intimately apposed to it, lies the nucleus vagi motorius dorsalis (f). The nucleus hypglossii (h) is separated from that of the vagus by the lightly stained nucleus intercalatus (g). Pre-hypoglossal (i), paracentral (j) and raphe (q) cell groups appear moderately stained, although dispersed by the longitudinal passing fibre systems. The nucleus ambiguus (o, and possibly, n) can also be seen as a densely stained group

Fig. 8. Medulla oblongata (approximately, stereotaxic plane P 10). The nucleus cuneatus medialis (a) has nearly disappeared at this level and is only represented by a few patches with positive AThChE stain, embedded within the most caudal portions of the vestibular complex (d). The nucleus cuneatus lateralis (b), shows a very pale AThChE stain. The descending nucleus of the trigeminal nerve (j) is irregularly stained and appears to be continuous with

medial longitudinal fasciculus. Its dorsolateral boundary can also be well outlined in view of the fact that the nucleus intercalatus (Fig. 7, in g) is less stained. According to Koelle (1952) this nucleus contains two kinds of cells: large and intensely stained, and medium sized, less well stained. The ventrolateral aspect of the nucleus is the only portion which is ill-defined. This appearance is in agreement with the image displayed in Golgi stained material where the dendrites of the nucleus are seen to extend in a ventrolateral direction to become intermingled with those of the cells of the adjacent parvocellular reticular formation. It is interesting that these darkly stained bands should follow the direction of the dendritic expansions rather than that of the fibres of the hypoglossal nerve which are more medially located. The nucleus prepositus hypoglossii (Fig. 2 V, in PO) lies medial to the caudal portion of the vestibular complex. If dendroarchitectonic criteria are used, this center is less extensive than usually accepted. It may correspond to a group of neurons that, like those of other specific precerebellar centers, display slightly wavy (allodendritic) dendrites.

The *nucleus supraspinatus* can be seen (S, in Figs. 1 I and 1 II), as a dark mass independant from the mass of the hypoglossal nucleus proper (NXII). If one regards the supraspinatus as a rostral continuation within the medulla of the medial groups of the anterior horn of the cervical spinal cord, the so-called somatic motor column of the medulla cannot be regarded with certainty as the representative of the anterior horn of the spinal cord.

The *nucleus abducens* (N VI in Fig. 3 IX) is easily recognizable in view of its location around the genu of the facial nerve which forms a pale and sharply

a dark band (i) that reaches the most ventral regions of the nucleus cuneatus medialis (h). The latter is separated from the solitary complex (f) by a pale region (g). The nucleus subtrigeminalis (k) is well stained. The nucleus ambiguus (l) appears very clearly outlined against the non-stained reticular core (o). Ventrolateral to it, lies a slightly stained region (m) of obscure significance

Fig. 9. Medulla oblongata (approximately, plane P 8). The most superficial layers of the dorsal cochlear nucleus (d), the striae acusticae (a) and a medial limiting borderline for the dorsal cochlear nucleus (c) appear to be the only regions related to the auditory pathway that stain intensely. The pars interpolaris of the nucleus of the trigeminal nerve is more densely stained in its medial component (e) than in its lateral portion (f). The facial nucleus (g) is intensely stained. The corpus pontocuneatus (b) appears as a darkly stained wedge between the descending root of the trigeminus and the restiform body

Fig. 10. Pons (approximately, stereotaxic plane P 7). The lower portion of the field is occupied by the strikingly pale, superior olivary complex (f). The abducens nucleus (a) is well stained. The nucleus of the trapezoid body shows a positive reaction in a restricted area (d). Some positively stained areas (b) may represent aberrant portions of the descending trigeminal nucleus. Dorsal to the olivary complex lies a densely stained band (c) of obscure significance

Fig. 11. Mesencephalon (approximately, plane A 4). The nucleus oculomotorius principalis (a) appears intensely stained. The red nucleus is irregularly stained. Its most medial portion (e) remains pale and is mostly made out of the fibres of the brachia conjunctiva. The central portion contains some slightly stained islands (c and d) separated by pale areas which do not show any constant pattern of distribution. The tegmentum pararubralis (see Fig. 5 XIX; TGPAR) remains pale, except for a small area, dorsolateral to the red nucleus (b)

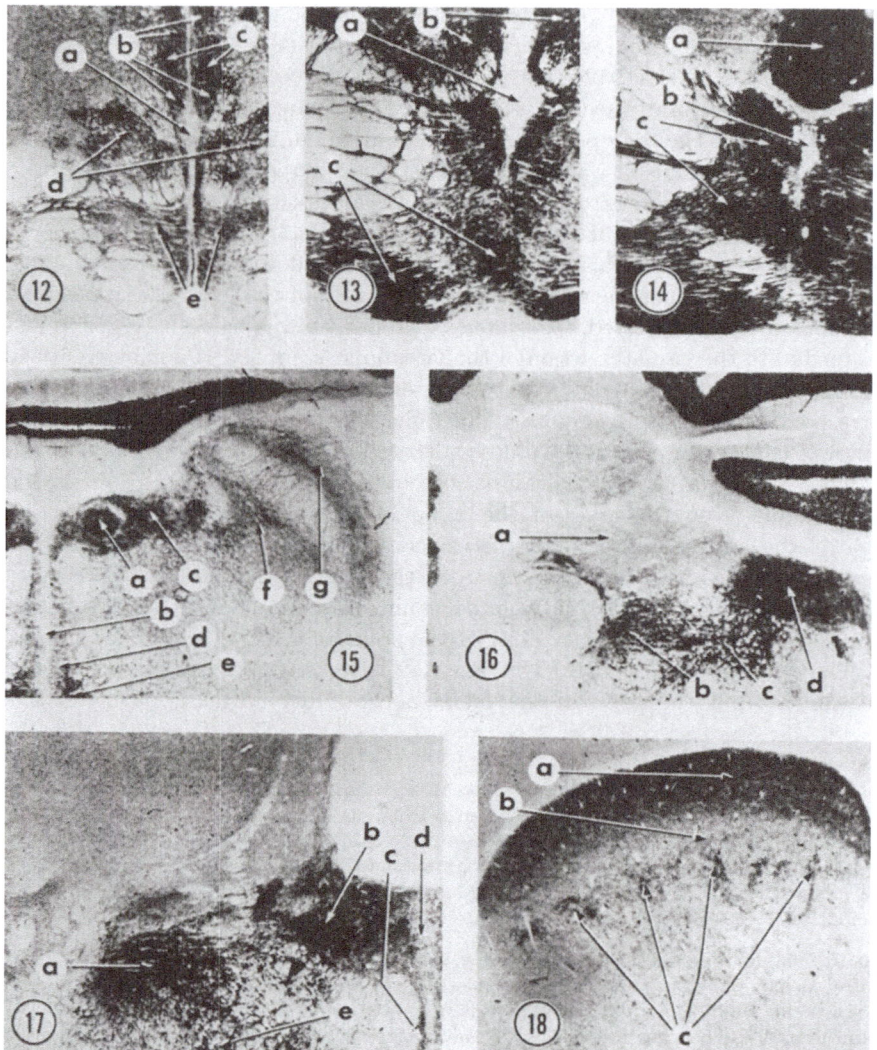

Fig. 12. Pons (approximately, plane P 4). In this section the processus supralemniscalis (d), together with certain densely stained islands (c) embedded within the nucleus centralis superior (b) constitute a symmetrically arranged center: the nucleus papilliformis. It shows the same intense coloration of the more ventrally located pontine nuclei (e)

Fig. 13. Pontine region (approximately, plane P 2). In the midline, a region rich in sagittal fibres (a) stands out as non-stained structure within the dark masses of the ventral nucleus papilliformis (b), or processus supralemniscalis. and the pontine nuclei (c)

Fig. 14. Rostral pontine region (approximately, plane A 2). In addition to the pontine nuclei (c), the nucleus interpeduncularis (a) stands out as one of the most densely stained nuclei within the brain stem

Fig. 15. Rostro-dorsal pontine region (approximately, plane P 4.5). The subventricular region appears well stained with a lateral, diffuse, griseum centrale (c), and a more medial, round and circumscribed, center, the dorsal tegmental nucleus of Gudden (a). In the median region, the nucleus centralis superior shows a median non-stained portion (b), a more lateral dark

outlined structure within it. In AThChE material it forms part of an intensely stained mass which includes the nucleus abducens proper, as well as two other centers of probably different significance: the nucleus retroabducens (Fig. 2 VI, in a) and the nucleus preabducens (Fig. 3 X, in a). These two centers are also intensely stained and, in AThChE material, no clearcut boundary can be established between them and the n. abducens. However, in Nissl and Golgi materials, one can see that they are made out of entirely different cells. The *nucleus retroabducens* (Fig. 2 VI, in a) corresponds to the rostral part of the classical nucleus prepositus hypoglossii. However, we are inclined to regard the latter as less extensive than usually accepted (Fig. 2 V, in PO). The *nucleus preabducens* (Fig. 3 X, in a) is a diffusedly organized region, populated by neurons entirely comparable to those of the griseum centrale (leptodendritic type). This center should not be confused with Gudden's nucleus tegmentosus dorsalis (Fig. 15, in a) which is a relatively well outlined structure within the griseum centrale, and rostral to the preabducens.

In Snell's paper (1961) the *nucleus trochlearis* can be seen as a very dark mass lying ventral to the griseum centrale and dorsolateral to the fibres of the medial longitudinal fasciculus (Snell's illustration 18). In AThChE stained sections it has a medial portion made out of cells interposed between the fibres of the medial longitudinal fasciculus and a lateral portion which is homogeneously stained. This lateral portion is the last one to disappear as one follows the nucleus in an orocaudal sequence. In Fig. 5 XVIII, the nucleus (NIV) can be seen as a relatively well outlined dark mass in contrast to the pale adjacent griseum centrale which at this level is poor in AThChE. More rostrally (Fig. 5 XIX) the median portion of the latter is darker and the separation becomes more difficult. The nucleus trochlearis should not be confused with any of the tegmental nuclei of Gudden, which are located more caudally, where the plane of the section encroaches upon the most caudal portion of the inferior colliculus and the lingula of the cerebellum.

region (d) which probably represents the centralis superior, sensu strictu, and some densely stained islands (e) which may correspond to the nucleus papillioformis. The pars dorsolateralis (g) and ventromedialis (f) of the caudal tegmentum peribrachialis appear relatively pale at this level

Fig. 16. Rostro-dorsal pontine region (approximately, plane P 3). The tegmentum cuneiformis (see TGCU in Fig. 4 XIII) constitutes a small wedge-shaped region that lies caudal and ventral to the inferior colliculus (a). It appears as a very pale region that becomes replaced rostrally by the intensely stained tegmentum suprabrachialis (b and c). In this plane, the griseum centrale appears also very dark

Fig. 17. Suprabrachial region and adjacent centers (approximately, plane P 2). The suprabrachial tegmentum (a) is characterized by strong stainability which becomes less intense as a result of the presence of the passing fibres of the brachium conjunctivum (e). The griseum centrale shows a densely stained lateral zone (b) and a pale median zone (d). The raphe contains some darkly stained spots (c)

Fig. 18. Superior colliculus. The stratum zonale and stratum griseum superficiale (a), appear intensely stained and separated from the stratum griseum profundum (c) by the pale stratum medullare intermedium (b). The stratum griseum profundum (c) is characterized by isolated "islands" rather than by a uniform stain

The *nucleus oculomotorius* (NIII, in Fig. 5 XX) can be seen as a dark wedge interposed between the fibres of the ventrally located medial longitudinal fasciculus. Caudally it becomes continuous with a dark region, equally interposed between the fibres of that fasciculus, which extends as far as the nucleus trochlearis. This dark region extends, dorsally, into the median griseum centrale of the mesencephalon and, ventrally, into the raphe region. It is not possible at this stage to determine whether or not it contains somatic motoneurons. On the other hand, the equally dark median region of the oculomotor wedge includes the nuclei of Perlia and Edinger-Westphal which, supposedly, contain autonomic motoneurons. Thus, the possibility exists that this median region, caudal to the oculomotor nucleus, may also be related to the autonomic parasympathetic efferent pathway for the eye.

The richness in AThChE appears to be even greater in *the autonomic motor centers* of the brain stem. Iijima *et al* (1969) have found that the dorsal motor nucleus of the vagus contains both, specific and non specific cholinesterases, although the former appears to be preponderant. This circumstance could be interpreted as significant and related to the fact that the vagus is a cholinergic nerve. Such significance is, however, less evident if one takes into account that there are so many other regions within the central nervous system that also show an intense AThChE stain. In Fig. 7, perhaps as a result of a certain degree of enzyme diffusion, the borderlines between the components of the dorsal vagal complex and neighboring structures are difficult to visualize. The dorsal motor nucleus (f) and the area postrema (e) appear to form a single evenly stained dark mass. The nucleus solitarius (c) also participates in this complex, although it is slightly paler. Medially, the nucleus intercalatus (g) stands out as a relatively unstained structure and, laterally, a very pale region (b) separates this complex from the nucleus gracilis (a). This pale band could represent the most caudal portion of the "nucleus" vestibularis medialis. A better control of diffusion artefacts would be necessary to furnish a more detailed analysis of this area. Following a modification of the AThChE technique which greatly reduces enzyme diffusion, Shute and Lewis (1960) were able to localize the salivatory center on the medial aspect of the genu of the facial nerve. By combining the AThChE technique with operative procedures leading to retrograde degeneration, a precise demarcation of the dorsal motor nucleus of the rat has been achieved by Lewis *et al.* (1970). It is interesting that, according to Koelle (1952) the dorsal motor nucleus of the vagus in the rat displays a low acetylcholinesterase activity, as opposed to what seems to be the case in the cat. This could be due to species differences which have already been shown to be quite remarkable (Friede, 1966).

Sensory Relay Centers and Neighbor Regions

Little correlation can be established between the hodological order of the sensory relay centers and their enzyme activity. For example, the principal and spinal trigeminal nuclei show high acetylcholinesterase content whereas the ventral cochlear nucleus, which is also believed to be a secondary sensory center, shows very little content. In the case of the vestibular nuclei, the area which shows the highest enzyme activity does not correspond to the distribution of the afferent fibres as described by Brodal *et al.* (1962).

There are only two trends that deserve being pointed out. The first one regards the secondary sensory centers which, with the exception of the cochlear and vestibular nuclei, are rich in enzyme (nucleus principalis and spinalis of the trigeminal nerve, nuclei gracilis and cuneatus medialis, dorsal horn of the spinal cord, and nucleus of the fasciculus solitarius). The superficial layers of the superior colliculus, i.e., the ones receiving a massive projection from the retina, are also intensely stained. The other trend regards the auditory pathway which, with the exception of the granular layer of the dorsal cochlear nucleus, is made out of centers which contain less enzyme than most other brain stem territories (ventral cochlear nucleus, deeper layers of the dorsal cochlear nucleus, superior olivary complex, nucleus trapezoideus medialis, nucleus of the lateral lemniscus and inferior colliculus). As regards the thalamic centers, ist should be noted that the geniculatus lateralis es extremely rich in enzyme, whereas the posteroventral group, and the geniculatus medialis, contain only a few scattered positively stained areas.

The *nucleus cuneatus medialis* (CM in Figs. 1 I through 1IV) displays an intense acetylcholinesterase stain, in contrast to the cuneatus lateralis. In its most caudal portion, the stain is more intense dorsally, whereas in its rostral portion the deep layers of the nucleus are also intensely stained. At this rostral level, there is a darkly stained mass, the nucleus supratrigeminalis (Fig. 1 IV, in Q) which forms sort of a bridge of densely stained material leading to the equally darkly stained spinal nucleus of the trigeminus. In view of the fact that both the cuneatus medialis and the trigeminalis spinalis are prethalamic sensori-somatic nuclei, the possibility that this region may constitute a prethalamic center must also be considered. In Golgi stained material, the most rostral pole of the nucleus cuneatus medialis can be easily differentiated from the caudal vestibular area if one takes into account the entirely different dendroarchitectonic patterns of these two regions (Ramon-Moliner, 1968). In AThChE stained material this is also possible in view of the fact that the vestibular complex (Fig. 7, in b) is considerably less intensely stained than the cuneatus medialis (Fig. 7, in a).

The *nucleus gracilis* (GR in Figs. 1 I, 1 II, and 1III) extends dorsally on each side of the midline, from the most caudal portion of the medulla to the level of the caudal pole of the "nucleus" vestibularis inferioris. In Nissl, in Golgi, and in AThChE materials, it is associated with the nucleus cuneatus medialis from which it can be easily outlined only in its most caudal portion. At that level, the nucleus lies close to the midline and is separated from the contralateral one by the dorsomedian septum of the medulla. At more rostral levels, when the fourth ventricle becomes widened, the nucleus is displaced and lies lateral to the dorso-vagal complex. This center appears to be very rich in AThChE and its appearance is very similar to that of the nucleus cuneatus medialis. A high cholinesterase activity was also reported by Snell (1961) in the cells of these two centers which, in his illustrations, display the same arrangement in the form of irregular spots separated by lighter areas which become more preponderant in the ventral and medial portions of the complex. Snell also illustrated, although he did not discuss it, the band of non stained material which separates the cuneatus-gracilis complex from the hypoglossal nucleus and which is regarded here as the most caudal extension of the vestibular complex (Fig. 7, in b).

The *nucleus tractus spinalis trigemini* (SV in Figs. 1 II through 2 VIII extends from the caudal pole of the nucleus principalis, at the rostral pontine level, to the most caudal portion of the medulla oblongata where it appears to become continuous with the dorsal horn of the cervical spinal chord. In a rostro-caudal sequence it has been subdivided (Olszewski, 1954) into three main portions: oralis, interpolaris, and caudalis. In addition, the pars caudalis (SV in Fig. 1) is usally subdivided into a subnucleus gelatinosus and a subnucleus magnocelluaris not clearly distinguishable in AThChE material. In this material the best outlined portions are the pars oralis and the pars caudalis. The pars interpolaris (SV in Fig. 2) is less conspicuous. The pars caudalis constitutes a mass as large as or even larger than the nucleus principalis. It is intensely stained and well outlined, even on its most medial border, which in Nissl and Golgi materials is slightly diffuse (Ramon-Moliner, 1968). A densely stained mass, the nucleus supratrigeminalis, (Figs. 1 III and 1IV, in Q) bridges the space between the cuneatus medialis and the spinalis trigemini. From the dendroarchitectonic point of view the cells of this region are generalized and can be compared to those of the deeper layers of the nucleus cuneatus medialis and those of the medial or magnocellular partion of the trigemini spinalis. The pars interpolaris, although not as massive as the pars caudalis, can still be seen as a dark mass medial to the descending tractus of the trigeminal nerve. From the dendroarchitectonic point of view, this portion differs drastically from the other two in that it contains generalized nerve cells comparable to those of the adjacent reticular formation. Thus, the presence of a high enzyme content throughout the length of the trigemini spinalis cannot be easily correlated with dendroarchitectonic patterns.

The *nucleus principalis trigemini* (PV in Figs. 3 IX and 3 X) lies caudal to the tegmentum entobrachialis and rostral to the "nucleus" vestibularis superior. It is wedged between the brachium conjunctivum, the brachium pontis, and the nucleus masticatorius which lie respectively dorsally, laterally and ventromedially (PV in Figs. 3 IX and 3 X). The fibres of the trigeminal nerve separate it form the nucleus masticatorius. Its anterior pole becomes continuous with the mesencephalic root which, following the medial edge of the brachium conjunctivum, extends to the mesencephalon. Its caudal pole is displaced ventrally and becomes continuous with the pars spinalis. In AThChE material, this center is very intensely stained, in contrast to the caudal tegmentum entobrachialis which lies rostral to it, and the vestibular complex which lies caudal to it. In our material it was not possible to distinguish any subnuclei, on the basis of their AThChE content.

The *nucleus nervi trigemini mesencephalicus* is made out of nerve cells apparently devoid of dendrites and is usually regarded as equivalent to the cells of the posterior root ganglia. It extends from the level of the caudal portion of the posterior commissure to the rostral pole of the nucleus masticatorius. It does not constitute a well delimited center in view of the fact that its cells are embedded in a matrix made out of overlapping dendrites of cells belonging to adjacent territories, and of passing ascending and descending fibres. In AThChE material it is difficult to ascertain whether or not these neurons are intensely stained in view of the fact that they are interposed between regions which are either moderately or intensely stained: the griseum centrale and the nucleus entobrachialis. At more rostral levels (see Fig. 5, XVII), where both the griseum centrale and the adjacent tegmentum (infracollicularis) are poorly stained, this nucleus cannot be identified either.

The *nucleus of the solitary tract* (e, in Fig. 1 IV) shows a slightly pale central region (Fig. 7, c) surrounded by a darker peripheral ring. Ventrolateral to it lie the fibres of the fasciculus solitarius (Fig. 7, d). In the most caudal portion of the medulla, the nucleus (Fig. 1 IIIa) lies medial and ventral to the nucleus gracilis, (Fig. 1 III, in GR) which is also densely stained. At more rostral levels it is separated from this somatic sensory center by the already mentioned lighter band which could represent the most caudal extension of the "nucleus" vestibularis inferioris (Fig. 7, in b). The dorsal visceromotor nucleus of the vagus and the nucleus of the solitary tract constitute, both in Golgi and in AThChE materials, a complex in which no clear separation can be established between the two components. In Nissl material, the separation is not very evident either, although the medioventral portion, where the viscero-motor neurons lie, is more densely packed with neurons of slightly larger size than those of the lateral or viscerosensory portion. In the most caudal level of the medulla the two nuclei of the solitary tract become inited in the midline by means of a bridge which lies dorsal to the central canal (Fig. 1 III, in c) to form the nucleus commissuralis (Ramon y Cajal, 1911).

The *colliculus superioris* (SCO in Figs. 5 XVII through 5 XX) can be roughly subdivided into four layers from the subpial region to the periventricular central gray matter. The most superficial layer (Fig. 18, in a) corresponds to the classical stratum zonale and stratum griseum superficiale and is characterized by high AThChE activity with a decreasing gradient in its ventral portion. The second layer (Fig. 18, in b) corresponds to the classical stratum opticum and stands out very clearly as a pale band. In all likelihood, it is mostly made out of preterminal optic fibers (Ramon y Cajal, 1911). Its borders are ill-defined, although the one which separates this layer from the superficial layer is much more evident than the ventral one. In AThChE material, the third layer corresponds to the classical strata griseum intermedium and medullare intermedium (Fig. 18, in c). Both have a characteristic uneven distribution of the stain with regularly spaced dark masses separated by a light stained background. The fourth layer, which is very pale, corresponds to the classical strata griseum profundum and medullare profundum. They cannot be delimited from the adjacent diffuse tegmentum infracollicularis but are well separated from the griseum centrale, which is slightly more darkly stained (Figs. 5 XVIII and 5 XIX).

The so-called *vestibular nuclei* (VL and VM in Figs. 2 V, 2 VI, and 2 VII) display such remarkable hodological and dendroarchitectonic similarities with the reticular formation that we are inclined to regard them as a portion of the latter (Ramon-Moliner and Nauta, 1966). The only difference would lie in the fact that a restricted portion of this mass receives sensory fibres from the peripheral vestibular apparatus. On the other hand, this area shares with the reticular formation a number of characteristics: cytological polymorphism; generalized dendrites, that is, long, radiating, and relatively rectilinear, extending into the adjacent territories; and absence of clearcut borderlines. Both in Nissl and Golgi stained materials, the demarcation of the vestibular complex from the adjacent reticular formation is totally arbitrary. In addition, *the vestibular complex shares with the reticular formation the fact that it has very heterogeneous*, both efferent and afferent. In AThChE material, two main subdivisions can be established: the lateral vestibular "nucleus" which, on the whole, stands out as relatively pale, probably as a result of the presence of numerous passing myelinated fibres, and the medial vestibular "nucleus", which is slightly more darkly stained. If priority is given to chemoarchitectonic characteristics, the nucleus vestibularis inferior should be regarded as smaller than usually accepted. It would correspond to a very pale band which is interposed between the nucleus cuneatus medialis and the solitary-vagal complex (Fig. 1 IV, in a). On the other hand, in AThChE material the "nucleus" vestibularis superior would appear to be the most rostral continuation of the "nucleus" vestibularis medialis at the rostral level of the 4th ventricle into which it protrudes as a dark mass (Fig. 2, VIII, in a).

As opposed to other sensory pathways, the *auditory system* is made out of several nuclei staggered allong the brain stem, It is doubtful, however, that these centers should constitute censecutive relay stations. In all probability, the majority of the neurons of the dorsal and ventral cochlear nuclei are secondary sensory and, if the same pattern established for other sensory pathways is applicable to the auditory one, the neurons of the cochlear nuclei should receive fibres from the peripheral neurons of the cochlear ganglion and project to the medial geniculate body. If so, the remaining centers (superior olivary complex, nucleus trapezoidalis, nucleus of the lateral lemniscus, and inferior colliculus) could constitute a pathway for collateral integration. It is interesting that all these centers are populated by specialized, allodendritic, neurons (Ramon-Moliner and Nauta, 1966; Ramon-Moliner, 1968) and that, both in Golgi and in AThChE materials, they constitute structures well segregated from the matrix of the reticular formation.

The *nucleus cochlearis dorsalis* can be easily subdivided into inner, intermediate and outer zones (d, e, and f in Fig. 2 VI). It constitutes an elongated and flattened mass applied to the lateral aspect of the corpus restiformis, and more caudally situated than the ventral cochlear nucleus. In AThChE material, the outer cellular zone is very darkly stained (Fig. 2 VI, in d; Fig. 2 VII, in c; Fig. 2 VIII, in c). Dorsally, this layer becomes continuous with the equally darkly stained striae acusticae dorsales. In the deeper layers of this center the AThChE stain is less intense. The outermost layer is very rich in glia and the possibility cannot be excluded that the intense stain could be due to the presence of non-specific cholinesterase. The same applies to an extremely narrow band of densely stained material (Fig. 2 VI, in c; Fig. 2 VII, in e) which separates the dorsal from the ventral cochlear nuclei. However, in some of our Golgi stained series we were able to observe in this area certain nerve cells with sagittally flattened and highly specialized dendritic fields.

The *nucleus cochlearis ventralis* (cv in Figs. 2 VII and 2 VIII) is remarkable because it contains some of the most specialized dendritic patterns of the brain stem. It shows only a moderate AThChE stain. A subpial darkly stained band can be seen on its dorsal lateral aspect at rostral levels. However this band could represent the most rostral portion of the nucleus cochlearis dorsalis (the internal granular layer).

In AThChE material, the *superior olivary complex* (CSO in Figs. 2 VII through 3 IX) can be identified with the naked eye as a relatively round, non-stained structure. It constitutes a "closed" nucleus (Mannen, 1960), insofar as its neurons have dendrites which do not extend into the adjacent reticular formation but remain within the center. It is surrounded by a capsule of completely non-stained fibres. In Nissl and in Golgi materials some difficulty may be encountered in differentiating the most ventral and rostral portions of the facial nucleus from the caudal superior olivary complex. This is not the case in AThChe material in view of their sharply different staining properties. Thus, in Fig. 2, VI, ventral to the darkly stained nucleus facialis, one can see a pale region which becomes continuous at rostral levels with the superior olivary complex. The lack of AThChE in the superior olivary complex constitutes a surprising finding in view of the importance that certain authors have given to the olivo-cochlear bundle (Desmedt and La Grutta, 1957; Osen and Roth, 1949) which, supposedly, is rich in acetylcholinesterase. In Fig. 10 (in b and c) one can see certain islands of intensely stained material which, topographically, correspond to the area where such authors have placed the olivo-cochlear bundle. In our opinion, however, this identification necessitates further confirmation (see: Morest, 1968).

Adjacent to the superior olivary complex are the nuclei trapezoidalis lateralis and trapezoidalis medialis. Since, from the dendroarchitectonic point of view, they are entirely different the former will be described here as *superior paraolivary nucleus* (Z in Figs. 2 VII through 3 IX). This center envelopes the superior olivary complex on its dorsolateral and ventrolateral portions. It is considerable more darkly stained than the superior olivary complex, although not much more than the adjacent reticular formation. In AThChE material, it stands out because it appears as a dark wedge interposed between the lateral aspect of the superior olivary complex and the central auditory fibres entering the corpus trapezoideus. The superior paraolivary nucleus constitutes a complex region which. in Golgi material, is populated by neurons with relatively long and wavy dendrites which differ in appearance from those of the dorsally located reticular formation, as well as from those of the adjacent superior olivary complex. The *nucleus trapezoidalis* (medialis) can be easily identified in Golgi material, where it appears populated by highly specialized neurons, entirely comparable, from the dendroarchitectonic point of view, to the neurons of the rostral portion of the ventral cochlear nucleus. In AThChE material (Fig. 2 VII, in NT) it appears to show the same degree of stainability as that of the dorsally located reticular formation unless a dark region (Fig. 10, in d) which lies dorsal to it can be regarded as an extension of the nucleus. This does not deem to be endorsed by observations in Golgi material, which at that level does not show the characteristic tufted neurons of the nucleus trapezoidalis.

The *nucleus lemnisci lateralis* (NLL, Figs. 3 XI through 4 XIV) is formed by two subnuclei. The dorsal nucleus appears as an ovoid mass which lies ventral to the inferior colliculus and lateral to the tegmentum suprabrachialis. The ventral nucleus appears as a band stretching from the above to the lateral portion of the medial lemniscus. The fibres of the lateral lemniscus cover the nucleus on its lateral and its medial aspects. In AThChE material such fibres remain pale and form a sort of capsule that envelopes the center. In addition, some fibres appear within the matrix of the nucleus as non-stained islands. On the whole, the nucleus of the lateral lemniscus appears to be relatively poor in AThChE, particularly when compared with the medially situated peribrachial tegmental areas which, particularly at rostral levels, are darkly stained.

The *colliculus inferioris* (ICO, Figs. 4 XIII through 5 XVIII) stands out as a result of its pale stain in AThChE material. The only slightly stained portion is a dark band on its lateral aspect which lies medial to the superficially situated fibres of the lateral lemniscus and which, at rostral levels, becomes decomposed into a series of ventrolateral scattered islands. Ventromedially, the center shows the same degree of staining as that of the griseum centrale. However, a very thin white band marks the borderline with the latter. The *nucleus parabigeminalis* is a small center, intensely stained in AThChE material (U, Fig. 5) which, because of its location, could be related to the auditory pathway. Its most caudal portion is compact and well outlined. Rostrally, it becomes continuous with the equally densely stained tegmentum retrogeniculatus, of which it forms part. Dorsal to it lie the fibres of the brachium of the inferior colliculus.

Specific Precerebellar Centers

In this class, only those centers that are believed to project in an exclusive or preponderant manner to the cerebellum are included. The vestibular complex, which also projects to the cerebellum is excluded in view of the fact that it also sends numerous fibres to many other centers. The class of the specific precere-bellar centers is also characterized by a curious trend: the neurons have more or less wavy dendrites (Ramon-Moliner, 1968) particularly evident in the inferior olivary complex and, to a lesser extent, in all the other centers. No correlation appears to exist, however, between the AThChE content of these centers and their other common features. Thus, while the pontine nuclei are amongst the richest regions in enzyme, the lateral cuneate is very poor. On the other hand, the inferior olivary complex, remarkable for its cytological and dendroarchi-tectonic homogeneity, shows a very uneven enzyme distribution.

The *inferior olivary complex* (OIM, OIL, and OIP in Figs. 1 II through 2 I) displays, on the whole, a positive AThChE stain, so that the center stands out as a well outlined structure against the pale background of the reticular formation. The nucleus olivaris accessorius dorsalis (OIL) is, by far, considerably more stained than the rest of the complex, particularly in its most dorsal portion and caudal pole. The lateroventral portion of this subnucleus is paler and has a mottled appearance. The same applies to the other components of the inferior olivary complex, the nucleus principalis (OIP) and the nucleus accessorius medialis (OIM), which are characterized by a general grey background with a number of irregularly scattered dark spots. The fibrillary capsule that surrounds the olivary complex, as well as the hilus, stand out as a pale matrix devoid of enzyme. A high cholin-esterase activity was also reported by Snell (1961) in the inferior olivary complex and it is apparent that in his illustrations the dorsal accessory nucleus is, as in our material, more densely stained than the rest of the complex.

The *nucleus cuneatus lateralis* (CL in Figs. 1 III and 1 IV) appears slightly stained but considerably less than the adjacent cuneatus medialis. This is a valuable finding because it permits the differentiation of two nuclei that, both in Nissl and Golgi materials are difficult, if not impossible, to tell apart. In its most caudal portion it is embedded within the corpus restiformis. More rostrally, the nucleus becomes wedged between the corpus restiformis, on its lateral aspect, and the descending root of the trigeminal nerve, on its medio-ventral aspect. Still more rostrally this wedge becomes continuous with Brodal's (1962) area X. There is a certain dendroarchitectonic similarity between the cells of area X and those of the corpus ponto-cuneatus. These two territories differ, however, in the fact that the corpus ponto-cuneatus is rich in enzyme.

The *corpus pontocuneatus* is a complex of discontinuous cell groups which extend in a relatively irregular manner, from the most rostrolateral portion of the lateral cuneate nucleus to the ventrolateral pontine cell groups (Ramon-Moliner, 1968). In spite of its discontinuity and the irregular size of its cells, it may constitute one single entity in view of the fact that its neurons are "allodendritic" and reminiscent of those found in the nucleus cuneatus lateralis and the pontine nuclei. In AThChE material these cell groups appear as a dark band which is first interposed between the corpus restiformis and the descending root of the trigeminus (Fig. 2 VI, in b), then medial to the cochlear complex (Fig. 2 VII, in f) and to the brachium pontis (Fig. 3 X, in d) to become, finally, continuous with the pontine nuclei as a lateral wedge visible in Fig. 3 XI, in c. The progression of the corpus ponto-cuneatus seems to reproduce the course followed by the neuroblasts that originate in the rhombic lip to migrate forwards and become pontine nuclei (Essick, 1907; Harkmark, 1954).

The *pontine nuclei* (PNT in Figs. 3 X through 5 XVIII) appear invariably well stained. As opposed to the olivary complex, the stain is equally intense for all the areas populated by nerve cells and only the presence of interposed fibres can account for the regions which are less dark. The fibres of the pyramidal tract appear as completely non-stained structures embedded and surrounded by the pontine grey matter. Snell (1961) pointed out that there is a very high cholinesterase activity around and between the descending motor fibres from the cerebral cortex, at the level of the pons. It is evident from his illustrations that he refers to the most caudal extension of the pontine nuclei which, at that level, surround the pyramidal tract. Thus, even though in the text he regards the enzyme content of the pontine nuclei as moderate, one must conclude from his illustrations that these centers were also intensely stained in his material. In their most caudal portion, the pontine nuclei extend laterally to form a wedge which lies medial to the middle cerebellar peduncle and becomes continuous, caudally, with the corpus ponto-cuneatus. On each side, one can see the accumulation of fibres of the middle cerebellar peduncle, pale but not as much as those of the pyramidal tract. This fibre system is supposed to contain a number of fibres which stain in AThChE material (Shute and Lewis, 1965). In their median portion, throughout their caudo-rostral extent, the pontine nuclei are interrupted by a pale sagittal band (Fig. 12, in a; Fig. 13, in a; and Fig. 14, in b). Rostrally, the pontine nuclei become condensed into a medio-ventral non-trabeculated mass, dorsal to which lies the nucleus interpeduncularis.

The *nucleus papillioformis* (Olszewski, 1954) probably represents a dorsally displaced portion of the pontine nuclei (PP in Figs. 3 XI through 4 XIV). It is formed of two paired supralemiscal masses (Fig. 12, in d) and certain median islands embedded in a slightly lesser stained matrix formed by the nucleus centralis superior (Fig. 12, in c). In Golgi stained material, both the supralemniscal region and the islands can be recognized as different from the adjacent territories because of their specialized dendritic patterns. Like the pontine nuclei, they are very rich in AThChE.

The *nucleus of the lateral funiculus* (nucleus "reticularis" lateralis) appears more stained than the adjacent reticular formation. This center (NFL in Figs. 1 II and 1 III) displays a typical trabeculated appearance which is more evident in its most caudal portion. At this level, it lies ventral to the descending root of the trigeminus, dorsolateral to the inferior olivary complex, and medial to the considerably paler adjacent reticular formation. On the whole, the nucleus is not as intensely stained as the more medially located inferior olive. However, it contains a few densely stained spots, particularly below the pial surface. In Golgi material (Ramon-Moliner, 1968) the nucleus is made out of a mixed population of neurons varying in the degree of specialization of their dendritic trees. The regions richer in acetylcholinesterase seem to correspond to those areas where the most specialized nerve cells are found. At more rostral levels the nucleus could be represented by two regions, one ventrolateral to the nucleus ambiguus, and the other ventral to the spinal root of the trigeminus (Fig. 8, in m and k). The latter is usually described as nucleus subtrigeminalis and contains nerve cells with a relatively specialized dendritic pattern.

The prehypoglossal and paramedian nuclei appear very well illustrated in Snell's paper (1961) as a trabeculated system made out of cells rich in enzyme, interposed between the non-stained pararaphal fibre bundles. These nuclei appear less stained but, nevertheless, evident in the material here studied (Fig. 7, in i and j). Snell reported a high enzyme content in the caudal reticular formation but he was referring, in all likelihood, to this precerebellar system.

Other Well Outlined Centers

The *nucleus ruber* (RU in Fig. 5 XX) appears relatively well outlined in AThChE material, not because of its richness in the enzyme, but because of the presence of a capsule of non-stained fibres around it. The enzyme activity is very unevenly distributed (Fig. 11). The dorsolateral portion is more evenly stained although paler (Fig. 11, in b). The ventromedial portion is the most unevenly stained, with a tendency to show a medial and a lateral dark area separated by a white band which, in all likelihood, is made out of fibres of the brachium conjunctivum. For further details, the reader is referred to McLennan's work (1969).

The *substantia nigra* (NG in Figs. 5 XVII through 5 XX) is extremely rich in AThChE in its middle portion. Ventral to the red nucleus, it is relatively well delimited, with the exception of a dorsomedial trabeculated portion which lies ventrolateral to this nucleus, and which has been described by Berman (1968) as nucleus retrorubralis. Rostrally, the substantia nigra is poorly delimited on its ventral side where it has a ragged apearance as a result of the presence of certain positively stained fibres which are interposed between the fibres of the cerebral peduncle (Olivier *et al.*, 1970a). In acetylcholinesterase material the most caudal and lateral portion of the substantia nigra becomes continuous with an equally darkly stained area, the tegmentum retrogeniculatum.

Diffuse Reticular and Tegmental Regions

Many conscientious efforts have been aimed at parcellating the "reticular formation" on a hodological basis, i. e., according to the distribution of afferent and efferent connexions (see reviews by Brodal, 1958; Mehler, 1969). However, in spite of such reports, this author still feels that it is justifiable to use a generic term for this territory. No outstanding cytoarchitectonic or dendroarchitectonic differences can be invoked to differentiate the caudal portions of the reticular formation from the rostral ones (Ramon-Moliner and Nauta, 1966; Ramon-Moliner, 1967). On the other hand, it appears desirable to comply with present nomenclature trends and reserve the term, tegmentum, for the pontomesencephalic regions of the reticular formation while retaining the term, reticular, for the most caudal portions, within the medulla.

The *caudal reticular formation*, as opposed to the ponto-mesencephalic r. f., does not display any outstanding features in AThChE material. The classical subdivisions into dorsolateral and ventromedial regions or into parvocellularis magnocellularis and gigantocellularis (RFP, RFM, and RFG in Figs. 1 III through 3 X) are not represented by any conspicuous changes in the cholinesterase content. This region offers a homogeneous appearance with only minor regional variations in the degree of stainability that can be stated more in terms of gradients than in terms of sharp borderlines. In general, it appears medium or weakly stained. Only the ascending and descending fibre systems within the caudal pons and the medulla are more lightly stained and the cells of the reticular formation interposed within these systems are probably responsible for the trabeculated appearance of the background. A few densely stained areas can be identified within this vast territory but these are not typical reticular regions as they contain neurons with slightly specialized dendrites and with specific projections to the cerebellum: the raphe and pararaphal unclei (Fig. 7, in j), the nucleus of the lateral funiculus or lateral reticular "nucleus" (Fig. 1 III, in NFL), the para-hypoglossal region (Fig. 7, in i), and the nucleus subtrigeminalis. There are also some scattered areas which may represent portions of the nucleus ambiguous (Fig. 7, in o and n).

The term *tegmentum suprapontinus* (TGSP in Figs. 3 X through 4 XVI) is used here to describe a vast region within the pons that can be considered as the rostral continuation of the "nucleus" gigantocellularis of the medulla oblongata. The use of this term appears more appropriate than that of nucleus pontis to avoid the possible confusion with the entirely different pontine nuclei. From the cytological and dendroarchitectonic points of view, it can be compared to the other generalized regions usually described as mesencephalic reticular formation. Rostrally, the tegmentum suprapontinus becomes replaced by the tegmentum retrorubralis, which does not contain gigantic neurons. Otherwise, the transition between both regions is gradual and in AThChE material no borderline can be established between them. Thus, the tegmentum suprapontinus can be regarded as a portion of the reticular (isodendritic) core which extends from a vertical plane passing in front of the nucleus abducens and the superior olivary complex to another arbitrary parallel plane passing roughly through the middle portion of the inferior colliculus. Medially, it is bounded by a series of midline centers in the following caudo-rostral sequence: the nucleus tegmentosus centralis inferioris, the medial islands of the nucleus papillioformis, and the nucleus tegmentosus centralis superioris. In the same sequence, on its dorsolateral aspect the following nuclei are staggered: the nucleus masticatorius, the pars caudalis and entobrachialis of the peribrachial tegmentum, and the dorsal nucleus of the lateral lemniscus. Laterally, it is separated from the lateral exposed aspect of the brain stem by the ventral nucleus of the lateral lemniscus. Ventrally, it is bounded by the corpus trapezoideus and the superior olivary complex in its most caudal portion and, more rostrally, by the lateral "wings" of the nucleus papillioformis which are interposed between this tegmental region and the medial lemniscus. In AThChE material, the tegmentum suprapontinus appears relatively pale, although not as much as the capsule of the nucleus of the lateral lemniscus which lies lateral to it. In transverse sections passing throgh the caudal mesencephalon (Fig. 4XIV), it appears as two pale, round and large areas on each side of the midline.

The *tegmentum retrorubralis* (TGRR in Fig. 5XVII) which forms the rostral pole of the tegmentum suprapontinus, shares with the latter the same degree of stainability in AThChE material. The reason for describing it separately is merely a topographical one. It is bounded, dorsally, by the fibres of the brachium conjunctivum which separate it from the tegmentum suprabrachialis and the tegmentum retrogeniculatus. Ventrally, it comes in contact with the pyramidal tract and with the fibres of the lateral and medial lemnisci. Medially, it is bounded by the nucleus centralis superior and, laterally, by the tegmentum retrogeniculatus. Rostrally, it becomes wedged between the fibres of the brachia conjunctiva as they approach the midline to decussate. At this level, however, such fibres do not form a compact bundle so that the rostral boundary of the tegmentum retrorubralis is very ill-defined. This rostral pole is continuous, laterally, with the tegmentum pararubralis and, dorsally, with the tegmentum infracollicularis, which are regions equally diffuse and relatively poor in enzyme.

The term *tegmentum peribrachialis* refers to another diffuse ponto-mesence-phalic region which is related topographically to the fibres of the brachia conjunctiva, as they course towards their decussation at middle mesencephalic levels. It can be subdivided into (a) pars caudalis, (b) pars cuneiformis, (c) pars supra-brachialis, and (d) pars entobrachialis.

The *pars caudalis* (TGPBC in Fig. 3XI) surrounds the brachia conjunctiva at the point where they enter the dorsal aspect of the pons. It can be subdivided, in turn, into a pars caudalis dorsolateralis which rides on the lateral aspect of the superior cerebellar peduncle, and a pars ventromedialis which is interposed between this fibre system and the fibres of the mesencephalic root of the trigeminal nerve (see g and f in Fig. 15). Both regions can be regarded as relatively poor in enzyme, particularly when compared with the more medially located griseum centrale.

The *pars cuneiformis* (TGCU in Fig. 3XII and 4XIII) constitutes only a restricted portion of what is usually described as nucleus cuneiformis (Taber, 1961; Berman, 1968). It corresponds to a mass of cells that extends like a wedge along the ventral and caudal surface of the inferior colliculus, separating it from the brachium conjunctivum and the dorsal nucleus of the lateral lemniscus which lies ventral to it (Fig. 16, in a). It displays a slight AThChE stain, although not as intense as the more rostrally situated pars suprabrachialis.

The *pars suprabrachialis* (TGSB in Figs. 4 XIII through 5 XVII) corresponds to the most rostral portion of the nucleus cuneiformis in Taber's and Berman's nomenclature. It lies in front of the pars cuneiformis and, like this one, it forms a rather diffuse matrix which fills, so to speak, the space left between the inferior colliculus, which is dorsally situated, and the dorsal nucleus of the lateral lemniscus and the brachium conjunctivum, which are ventrally situated. However, unlike the pars cuneiformis, it is a region rich in AThChE. The brachium conjunctivum separates the pars suprabrachialis from the pars entobrachialis, which displays cytoarchitectonic, dendroarchitectonic and histochemical characteristics similar to those of the pars suprabrachialis. Therefore, these two rostral portions of the peribrachial tegmentum are considered here as separate entities only for topographical reasons. At more rostral levels, as the fibres of the brachium conjunctivum become more ventrally situated, the pars entobrachialis disappears while the suprabrachialis becomes enlarged. The pars suprabrachialis continues forward as far as the level of the decussation of the brachia conjunctiva, at which point it becomes replaced by the tegmentum infracollicularis. This one differs from the pars suprabrachialis in that it is very poor in enzyme. Medially, the pars suprabrachialis is continuous with the griseum centrale mesencephali which is also darkly stained.

For the topographical reasons above mentioned the *pars entobrachialis* (TGEB in Figs. 3 XII through 4 XIV) is only well-defined in its most caudal portion. This region can also be regarded as the most lateral extension of the tegmentum dorsomedialis mesencephali which is also rich in enzyme. Ventrally, it fades gradually and merges with the tegmentum suprapontinus.

In Golgi material the *tegmentum dorsomedialis mesencephali* (TGDM in Figs. 3 XII through 4 XV) appears to be very similar to the tegmentum suprapontinus and the tegmentum retrorubralis which lie ventral and lateral to it. In AThChE material the region constitutes a dark mass with diffuse borderlines which lies on each side of the medial longitudinal fasciculus. It should not be confused with Gudden's nucleus tegmentosus profundus, which is a small and well-outlined, allodendritic, center encased within the tegmentum dorsomedialis. Laterally, this region becomes continuous with the equally darkly stained tegmentum entobrachialis. Gudden's *nucleus tegmentosus profundus* lies on each side of the midline, ventrolateral to the medial longitudinal fasciculus and appears as a well-outlined mass both in Nissl and in Golgi materials (Ramon-Moliner, 1968). In AThChE material, however, it is difficult to differentiate it from the tegmentum dorsomedialis, within which it is encased.

The *tegmentum lateralis mesencephali* (TGLM in Figs. 4 XV and 4 XVI) is a relatively small region which lies under the exposed lateral aspect of the mesencephalon immediately in front of the nucleus of the lateral lemniscus, and caudal to the tegmentum retrogeniculatum. It lacks any remarkable histological or histochemical properties and shows poor AThChE staining. The reason why it deserves being coined as a separate region lies in that it differs, both from the nucleus of the lateral lemniscus which has an entirely different dendrochitectonic pattern, and from the tegmentum retrogeniculatus which is rich in enzyme. The tegmentum lateralis mesencephali can also be regarded as a caudolateral extension of the tegmentum retrorubralis.

The *tegmentum retrogeniculatus* (TGRG in Figs. 5 XVII and 5 XVIII) lies rostral to the previously described region and rostrolateral to the tegmentum retrorubralis. As opposed to the latter, it is darkly stained and is made out of two portions: a pars dorsalis, or compacta, and a pars ventralis or reticulata. The pars compacta corresponds, in part, to the nucleus sagulum (Berman, 1968; Taber, 1961). It extends further caudally than the pars ventralis and forms a densely stained spot (nucleus parabigeminalis) that lies dorsal to the tegmentum lateralis (in U, Fig. 5). The pars ventralis has diffuse characteristics and blends ventrally with the most caudolateral portions of the substantia nigra. In AThChE material all these centers are rich in enzyme and form a sort of mesencephalic collar or ring around the mesencephalon. Dorsally, this ring includes the griseum centrale; laterally, the tegmentum peribrachialis and retrogeniculatus; and, ventrally, the substantia nigra and the nucleus interpeduncularis.

The *tegmentum infracollicularis* (TGIC) in Fig. 5 XVIII, XIX, and XX) corresponds to the rostral and dorsal portion of Berman's central tegmental field. It lies ventrolateral to the deeper layers of the superior colliculus, lateral to the griseum centrale and dorsal to the tegmentum pararubralis, from which it is separated in the present account for purely topographical reasons. It is poor in enzyme, as opposed to the tegmentum suprabrachialis which lies caudally. It becomes continuous, at more rostral levels, with the tegmentum paracommissuralis, or "nucleus" of the posterior commissure. This last region (not illustrated) is equally poor in enzyme and shares with the rest of the tegmental areas very ill-defined borderlines.

The *tegmentum pararubralis* (TGPAR in Figs. 5 XVIII, 5 XIX, and 5 XX) constitutes the rostrolateral continuation of the tegmentum retrorubralis with which is shares practically identical cytoarchitectonic, dendroarchitectonic and histochemical characteristics. It lies dorsolateral to the red nucleus, dorsomedial to the lemniscus medialis, and ventral to the tegmentum infracollicularis. Rostrally it becomes continuous with the prerubral fields, in the subthalamus (not illustrated). The latter are not particularly rich in enzyme but considerably more so than the adjacent specific thalamic centers.

The *tegmentum paralemniscalis* (TGPL in Fig. 5 XX) corresponds to Berman's nucleus of the brachium of the inferior colliculus. It forms a wedge interposed between the ventrally located substantia nigra, the medial lemniscus (which in AThChE material stands out as a pale area medial to this tegmental region) and the ventral portions of the medial geniculate body which lie lateral to it.

The *tegmentum ventralis* (ventral tegmental area of Tsai) lies ventral to the red nucleus, lateral to the nucleus interpeduncularis or its afferent system, the fasciculus retroflexus, and caudal to the mammillary nuclei (TGV in Fig. 5 XX). When compared to other tegmental regions it may be regarded as rich in enzyme. However, it is not as rich as the adjacent nucleus interpeduncularis which constitutes, perhaps, the richest region in enzyme of the whole brain stem (Lewis *et al.*, 1967).

Midline and Paramedian Nuclei of the Brain Stem

It is not easy to establish a correspondence between the various midline regions as displayed in AThChE material and those that have been proposed on the basis of cell size, shape, and distribution of the Nissl substance. A detailed cytoarchitectonic analysis of the raphe nuclei of the brain stem of cat was carried out by Taber *et al.* (1960). However, the cytoarchitectonic picture does not seem to reflect any evident histochemical trends and, for this reason, no attempt will be made here to establish a strict correspondence with the nomenclature used by the above authors.

If one pays attentiation exclusively to the pattern of AThChE distribution, the following midline regions or centers can be delineated in a caudal to rostral sequence: the nucleus of the raphe of the medulla oblongata (which can be arbitrarily subdivided into pars dorsalis, profunda, and interolivaris); the nucleus tegmentosus centralis inferioris; the nucleus tegmentosus centralis superioris; the tegmentum dorsomedialis (which includes Gudden's nucleus tegmentosus profundus); the griseum centrale and related nuclei; and the nucleus interpeduncularis. The tegmentum dorsomedialis and the griseum centrale are described in other sections of this report (see: diffuse tegmental regions and subependymal regions). One should also bear in mind that the region of the raphe often contains sagittally running fibre systems with very few or no neurons interposed between them. When this is the case, the region of the raphe stands out in AThChE material as a strikingly pale midline structure.

The *nucleus of the raphe of the medulla oblongata* (NRM in Figs. 1 III, 1 IV, and 2 V) is probably not much more intensely stained than the nearby reticular formation. It lies strictly in the midline and should not be confused with the paramedian nuclei. It is made out of cells which occupy the interstices left between the fibres of the various medially descending tracts of the medulla oblongata which stand out, on each side, as non-stained structures. The pars dorsalis constitutes a trabeculated region, medial to the hypoglossal nuclei. Laterally, it becomes continuous with the adjacent paramedian nuclei. The pars profunda corresponds to Taber's nucleus raphe pallidus and can be seen in Fig. 1 IV as a darkly stained medial band. Further rostrally, at the level of the nucleus prepositus hypoglossii, it becomes dorsally displaced and lies interposed between the fibres of the medial longitudinal fasciculus (Fig. 2 V). The pars interolivaris corresponds to Taber's nucleus raphe pallidus and is less intensely stained than the two previous subdivisions.

In AThChE material, the *nucleus tegmentosus centralis inferioris* (CI, in Fig. 3 X) could be considered as the most caudal extension of the nucleus tegmentosus centralis superioris. However, it is studied here as a possibly different entity in view of the fact that it is often refered to as nucleus raphe pontis. In the plane illustrated in Fig. 3 X, it is formed by two darkly and evenly stained bands on each side of the midline. It is interesting that, caudal to this center, the midline region of the pons (Figs. 2 VI, 2 VII, and 2 VIII) does not display any outstanding features. Thus, the nucleus raphe magnus described by Taber cannot be identified at all in AThChE material.

The *nucleus tegmentosus centralis superioris* (CS in Figs. 3 XII through 5 XVII) is a sagittally flattened agglomeration of cells which continues rostrally the centralis inferioris. It extends as far as the caudal portion of the decussation of the brachia conjunctiva. In Nissl stained material it is not easy to establish the boundary between the centralis inferioris, the centralis superioris and the medial "islands" of the papillioformis. In Golgi material the situation is clarified to a certain extent. The nuclei centralis superioris and inferioris are made out of cells with rectilinear dendrites which have little tendency to branch and constitute a sort of matrix within which the islands of the nucleus papillioformis are embedded. The latter are characterized by cells with a specialized dendritic pattern very similar to that of the pontine nuclei. In view of the fact that these midline centers have a strong cholinesterase stain, the differentiation is not easy. In Fig. 12, the most caudal portion of the nucleus centralis superioris is seen in b, and it is possible that the darker regions seen in c, could correspond to displaced portions of the papillioformis.

The *nucleus interpeduncularis* constitutes one of the most intensely stained regions of the brain stem (IP in Fig. 5 and a in Fig. 14). It is a "closed" nucleus (Mannen, 1960), extremely well outlined from the adjacent structures, regardless of the technique used to study it. It is unpaired and lies in the midline, in the depth of the interpeduncular fossa, between the two cerebral peduncles. According to Lewis *et al.* (1967) it could be the richest region in AChE of the whole brain. It is ovoid in shape and its caudal pole is larger than the rostral one. The rostral pole remains well outlined, even though the adjacent ventral tegmental region of Tsai is also relatively well stained.

In the upper pontine region a median pale septum extends from the floor of the fourth ventricle to the ventrally located transversal fibres of the trapezoid body. At more rostral levels this septum becomes less outstanding on its dorsal portion (Figs. 3 XII through 4 XVI). It can be seen as a median pale straight line within the tegmental nuclei centralis inferioris and superioris. The most ventral portion of this median septum can be followed rostrally as a pale and very well outlined median structure as far as the ventral aspect of the nucleus interpeduncularis Fig. 14, in b).

Subependymal Regions

Generally speaking, these regions are poorly understood. Only a few are well outlined structures: the area postrema, the cubcommissural organ, the medial nucleus of the habenula and, with certain reservations, the nucleus prepositus hypoglossii. The remaining majority constitute a well outlined, non-stained core in myelin preparations. However, such sharp demarcation is lost in Golgi material, where the dendrites of neighboring territories are seen enter the subependymal layers as if a natural borderline of any kind existed between them. Berman (1968) has coined in his atlas a number of these subventricular and periaqueductal diffuse regions: the subependymal granular layer of the medulla and pons, the nucleus prepositus hypoglossii, the nucleus tegmentalis dorsalis, the nucleus coerulus, the nucleus incertus, the pontine gray matter, the periaqueductal gray matter, the nucleus interstitialis and the nucleus of Darkschewitch. In successful Golgi preparations, all these regions appear to share one common feature: they are populately by small neurons with scarce but long and relatively rectilinear dendrites which in previous communications have been described as "lepto-dendritic" (Ramon-Moliner, 1967, 1969). The hypothalamus is also populated by this neuronal type.

Within the category of the subependymal centers, the well outlined ones (the area postrema, the n. prepositus hypoglossii, the n. subcommissuralis, and the medial nucleus of the habenula) are well stained structures in AThChE material. The remaining diffuse ones display a considerable variation in the degree of stainability, often completely unrelated to any evident cytoarchitectonic characteristics.

In *area postrema* is located in the most caudal portion of the fourth ventricle. This territory os often confused with the adjacent nucleus of the solitary tract. At one time, it was regarded as a glial formation but, according to the work of Morest (1960), it contains not only glial but also neurons. In Nissl stained material the area is composed of densely aggregated small cells which have a very scarce amount of cytoplasm. This area forms an enlarged protuberance in the lateral wall of the fourth ventricle. Its cell density allows one to differentiate it from the adjacent nucleus of the solitary tract. In Fig. 7, in e, this territory cannot be clearly outlined from the adjacent solitary-vagal complex. Other authors have been more successful and have demonstrated a much more detailed parcellation of this area (Gwyn and Wolstercroft, 1968; Iijima and Bourne, 1968; Iijima et al., 1969; Lewis et al., 1970). In Golgi stained material one can see that the dendritic processes of the neurons of the solitary-vagal complex often penetrate the area postrema.

The *nucleus prepositus hypoglossii* (PO in Fig. 2 V) sensu latu, constitutes a mass of nerve cells and neuroglia on the dorsomedial region of the upper medulla oblongata, extending from the rostral pole of the nucleus hypoglossii to the caudal pole of the nucleus abducens. In our AThChE material it does not lend itself to any parcellation and it is not even possible to determine its borderlines with the two motor nuclei between which it is interposed. However, in Nissl material the separation is clear. In Golgi material, there appears to be a caudal portion (PO in Fig. 2 V) with small and slightly wavy dendrites which could correspond to the precerebellar center described by Brodal et al. (1962) as nucleus prepositus. Rostral to this small cell group, this subependymal structure is populated by leptodendritic neurons (Ramon-Moliner, 1967, 1969) comparable to those of the upper pontine griseum centrale. The nucleus abducens is interposed between these two structures. For this reason, pending further clarification, the terms *nuclei retroabducens* (a, in Figs. 2 VI and 2 VII) and *preabducens* (a, in Fig. 3 X) are suggested here. The other two well outlined subependymal derivatives, the subcommissural organ and the medial nucleus of the habenula, have not been illustrated in the present report. They are rich in AThChE.

The *griseum centrale pontis* can arbitrarily be subdivided into a caudal portion, which corresponds to the nuclei retroabducens and preabducens, and a rostral portion which lies on the floor of the fourth ventricle, immediately behind the caudal opening of the aqueduct. Medially, the rostral griseum pontinus surrounds a relatively well outlined center, the nucleus tegmentosus dorsalis of Gudden (Fig. 15, in a). Laterally, ut may correspond to the locus coeruleus (Fig. 15, in c) as outlined by Friede (1961) in cat, but not to that outlined by Olszweski and Baxter (1954) in man. All these regions show an intense AThChE stain.

The *griseum centrale mesencephali* surrounds the aqueduct. Caudally, it lies medial to the inferior colliculi, ventral to the intercollicular commissure and dorsal to the tegmentum dorsomedialis mesencephali. At this level, its ventral portion is positively stained (GC in Figs. 4 XIV, 4 XV and 4 XVI) Rostrally (Figs. 5 XVII through 5 XX), it becomes pale and only a median wedge interposed between the medial longitudinal fasciculi remains stained.

Discussion

1. Cholinergic Transmission in the Nervous System

The fact that acetylcholine is a transmitter at the muscle end plate seems now well established. There is also convincing evidence, from electron microscopic studies, that AChE or, at least, an enzyme that hydrolyzes AThChE, accumulates selectively in the folded subsynaptic apparatus of the muscle end plate (Brown, 1961; Zachs and Blumberg, 1961; Barrnett, 1962; Lewis and Shute, 1966).

In some territories within the central nervous system, acetylcholine also seems to play an important role, although the interpretation of this role is more elusive than in the case of the muscle end plate. The cholinoceptive nature of the Renshaw cells in the anterior horn of the spinal cord was demonstrated by Eccles *et al.* (1954, 1956) and Curtiss and Eccles (1958). These neurons are believed to be stimulated by collaterals arising from the axons of motoneurons and, in turn, exert an inhibitory influence on the motoneurons. They appear to be cholinoceptive, that is, sensitive to acetylcholine, but not cholinergic. In other words, their inhibitory action on motoneurons would not be mediated by acetylcholine. Erulkar *et al.* (1968) made an attempt to localize the Renshaw cells and believed that they lack any significant amount of acetylcholinesterase.

David *et al.* (1963) produced evidence supporting the cholinergic nature of the transmission at the level of certain synapses of the lateral geniculate body in the cat. They found that the injection of acetylcholine enhanced the postsynaptic geniculate response and believed that this was not the result of a direct effect on the geniculate neurons but rather on the afferent fibres. On the other hand, Curtiss and Davis (1963) had questioned the possibility that acetylcholine should be a transmitter in the lateral geniculate body. Curtiss and Crawford (1965) and Crawford *et al.* (1966) studied the effect of acetylcholine on the cerebellum and believed that acetylcholine acts directly on the Purkinje cells but questioned that this action could be done through the intervention of the granule cell pathway.

Following micro-injections of acetylcholine in the brain stem of cat, Cordeau *et al.* (1963) were able to detect EEG and behavioral changes suggesting that acetylcholine may be involved in the activation of consciousness. George *et al.* (1964) believed that there is a cholinergic mechanism involved in the induction of paradoxical sleep. The work of La Torre (1968) also seems to indicate that psychological factors may play an important role in the brain levels of acetylcholinesterase, such levels being significantly higher in animals placed in an enriched environment.

Thus, even though the exact site of action of acetylcholine in the complex synaptic arrangements of the central nervous system may be open to debate, the body of evidence points to the presence of cholinergic mechanisms. In addition, a parallel uneven distribution of the three elements involved in the cholinergic system (acetylcholine, cholineacetylase, and acetylcholinesterase) has been reported for a number of regions of the central nervous system. The following areas display an intense AChThE stain and have been shown to contain high levels of acetylcholine or cholinacetylase: the striatum (MacIntosh, 1941; Feldberg and Vogt, 1948; Hebb and Silver, 1956; McLennan, 1964; Fahn and Côté, 1968), the lateral geniculate body, the region of the hypoglossal nucleus and the dorsal complex of the vagus (Feldberg and Vogt, 1948), and the nucleus interpeduncularis (Lewis *et al.*, 1967).

2. The Significance of a Positive AThChE Stain

In view of the above, it would appear that the histochemical demonstration of acetylcholinesterase, either with biochemical or histochemical methods, would automatically demonstrate the cholinergic character of any given center of pathway. This conclusion, however, is not warranted. As pointed out by Silver (1967), "workers who invoke histochemical results to support results obtained by other techniques should be aware of the vagaries of histochemistry." There are a number of contradictory observations that are difficult to interpret on the basis of such a simple correlation. The cerebellum provides one of the most striking examples. This center, which in a number of species shows an intense acetylthiocholinesterase stain, has been reported to be poor in acetylcholine or cholineacetylase (MacIntosh, 1941; Feldberg, 1950; Feldberg and Mann, 1946; Feldberg and Vogt, 1948; Hebb and Silver, 1956; Hebb, 1955, 1961; Silver, 1967; Fahn and Côté, 1968). The same applies to the posterior roots and ganglia of the spinal cord which were reported to give a positive acetylthiocholine stain (Snell, 1961) and yet appear to be poor in cholineacetylase or acetylcholine (Feldberg and Vogt, 1948). Even more puzzling is the finding reported by Friede (1967) on the remarkable differences of acetylthiocholinesterase distribution according to the animal species under study. In the cat, the stain is quite strong in the granular layer while the molecular layer remains pale. In parakeet, the molecular layer is the one which stains strongly, while the granular layer remains pale. In the aquirrel monkey, none of the layers are stained, whereas in the red squirrel both layers are strongly stained. Friede and Fleming (1964) were led to conclude that "There is in the cerebellum a possible choice between a cholinergic or non-cholinergic type of transmission and ... either type of transmission can be used by a given species to operate the same circuit." This, however, is not so easy to accept. It is difficult to imagine how, in biological systems, a given set of circuits could at a given time of evolution change from cholinergic to non-cholinergic transmission. Furthermore, a positive AThChE stain has been found in well-established adrenergic sites (Koelle and Friedenwald, 1949; Koelle, 1955; Lewis and Shute, 1969).

The subsynaptic distribution of AThChE in motor end-plate is now generally accepted. But in the central nervous system only a few instances of parasynaptic

distribution have been reported (Lewis and Shute, 1966). The enzyme accumulates, instead, in the granular endoplasmic reticulum, within the perikaryon and
the initial portion of the dendrites, sometimes in the axolemma, underneath the
myelin sheath, that is, sites which are far removed from synaptic contact. The
occasional presence of a positive AThChE stain in the axolemma could endorse
Nachmansohn's theory (1964, 1970) on the role of acetylcholine in nerve conduction, but it still remains to be explained why most synaptic sites within the central
nervous system so seldom display an evident AThChE stain. In any case, a universal cholinergic mechanism for axonal conduction must be rejected on the basis
of the available electron microscopic evidence since the location of AThChE
underneath the axolemma appears to hold true only for a restricted number of
nerve fibres. Furthermore, such universal cholinergic transmission would be
difficult to reconcile with the fact that axons contain only the smooth type of
endoplasmic reticulum, and are practically devoid of the granular type, i.e., the
only structure which consistently appears to be rich in AThChE. It is interesting
that this enzyme should pile up in the proximal stump of severed axons (Shute
and Lewis, 1961), a circumstance which was used as a criterion to determine the
polarity of conduction in a number of fibre tracts (Shute and Lewis, 1963a,
1963b, 1965, 1967, 1969; Lewis and Shute, 1967; and Lewis *et al.* 1967). Thus,
retrograde neuronal degeneration appears to entail an accumulation of AThChE
in the axonal segment which remains continuous with the perikaryon, as well as
the long known phenomenon of chromatolysis within the latter. At present it is
not possible to prove that there is a significant relation between these two events,
but one cannot exclude the possibility that the changes in the granular endoplasmic reticulum associated with the phenomenon of chromatolysis could result
in a depletion along the severed axon of AThChE and other possible enzymes
originally confined to the perikaryon.

There is also the possibility that the esterases which hydrolyze ACh and
AThCh may not be as equivalent as generally believed. Koelle and Friedenwald (1949) had already mentioned that the amount of CO_2 liberated with AThCh
as substrate is greater than with ACh. On the other hand, it is long known that
AChE can be involved in non-conducting mechanisms since it is present in great
concentration in erythrocytes. In view of this, one cannot discard the possibility
that at least some of the areas which show an intense AThChE stain may not
necessarily correspond to sites where cholinergic transmission takes place.

It is important to bear in mind the fact that ACh constitutes only a very small
percentage of the normally occurring esters of choline of the brain. Lecithins and
sphingomyelins are lipids rich in choline and the brain may countain up to 45
per kg of these lipids (Spector, 1965; King and Sperri, 1961). In this respect, it
is interesting that the family of organophosphorous compounds includes anticholinesterase agents, as well as demyelinating ones (Barnes and Denz, 1953).
Furthermore, acetylcholine itself could be involved in activities other than those
implicated in nervous transmission. The experiments of Hokin and Hokin (1956)
showed that the turnover of certain phospholipid compounds is increased when
acetylcholine is applied either to brain tissue, submandibular and parotid sali-
vary glands, or pancreas. Consequently, its hydrolysis by cholinesterase may often
have a role totally unrelated to nervous conduction. Conversely the so-called

non-specific cholinesterase, butyryl cholinesterase, pseudo-cholinesterase, or serum cholinesterse, cannot be excluded from nervous conduction (Desmedt and La Grutta, 1957). On the other hand, it appears that there are several types of serum cholinesterase (Whittaker, 1969) and, by the same token, it is possible that there should be several enzymes capable of hydrolysing AThCh. There are also many neuronal groups which are rich in pseudo-cholinesterase (Ord and Thomson, 1952; Cavanagh et al., 1954; Cavanagh and Holland, 1961; Foldes et al., 1962; Roessmann and Friede, 1966; Friede, 1967; Lewis and Flumerfelt, 1970) so that the notion that this enzyme is confined to glia and capillaries no longer holds true.

In conclusion, when confronted with a positively stained region, one should bear in mind that several interpretations are possible. Indeed, the region may be cholinoceptive, i. e., it may constitute a *target* for a neural ACh releasing system involved in nervous conduction (Wurzel, 1967). But to warrant this conclusion it would be necessary to prove that the enzyme that acts on AThCh does not hydrolyse other normal substrates which may not necessarily be related to synaptic or nervous conduction. It is doubtful that mere resistance to certain inhibitors like eserine or DFP should provide a reliable control, particularly if one takes into account that the brain contains relatively large amounts of sphingomyelins and lecithins which are complex esters of choline that are considerably more abundant than ACh. For this reason, one must regard with suspicion the value of the present histochemical techniques to determine the cholinergic character of any given center or pathway. As yet, this can be done only with biochemical techniques capable of demonstrating the presence of either ACh, or ChA or else, by iontophoresis, to determine the specific sensitivity to ACh.

Summing up, the observer of histochemical material must not: (a) forget that AThCh is not a natural substrate and that, even though its esterase may be identical to AChE, this is not completely proven; (b) overlook the fact that what determines the cholinergic character of a given structure is not the presence of AChE but that of its substrate, ACh, and that this substance is not "stainable"; (c) take for granted that an intense stain indicates a region where greater synthesis or release of ACh takes place; (d) forget that a strong stain merely indicates that, if acetylcholine is released there, it will be readily destroyed; (e) regard non-stained structures as necessarily non-cholinergic, as they may still contain ACh destined to be conducted along axons and hydrolysed elsewhere.

3. The Distribution of Acetylthiocholinesterase in the Brain Stem

The Non-Stainability of Fibre Bundles. The general impression gained from the study of our series is that, in general, fibre bundles within the central nervous system are not stained with Koelle and Friedenwald's (1949) AThChE technique. This does not necessarily mean that such bundles should be devoid of AThChE, but it certainly seems to indicate that their esterase content is considerably less significant than that found in territories where nerve cells are present. This impression is at variance with the report by Shute and Lewis (1961, 1963a, 1963b, 1965), on the presence of cholinesterase containing fibre systems in the hind brain. It must be pointed out, nevertheless, that in the present work no lesions were placed and no attempt was made to trace pathways or establish the polarity of their conduction.

The non-stainability of fibre systems could be attributed to the lipids of the myelin sheath that could constitute a barrier fot the access of the various chemicals used in the technique (Nachmansohn, 1970). If this was the case, one could expect that the fibre bundles that run parallel to the plane of the section would show greater resistance to the stain than the ones that are cut transversely. However, with one single exception to be mentioned below, all compact bundles, whether transversely or longitudinally cut, appeared extremely pale in the material studied. Amongst the fibre bundles that were cut transversely and that stand out as remarkably well outlined pale structures, the following can be mentioned: the pyramidal tract, the medial longitudinal fasciculus, the tectospinal tract, the medial lemniscus, the brachia conjunctiva, the descending root of the trigeminal nerve, as well as all the ascending and descending fibre systems in the dorsal, lateral and ventral funiculi, at the level of the most caudal medulla oblongata. Amongst the fibre systems which are also conspicuous as pale structures and made out of fibres running parallel to the plane of the section, the following can be mentioned: the brachium pontis, the fibres of the corpus trapezoideus, the fibres of the lateral lemniscus as they bend to reach the inferior colliculus, the fibres of the dorsal spino-cerebellar tract as they bend dorsally to reach the inferior cerebellar peduncle (corpus restiformis) and the fibres of the decussation of the brachia conjunctiva and of the intercollicular commissure.

In addition to the above mentioned fibre systems there are others not so well outlined but, nevertheless, conspicuous. This applies to the efferent fibres of most motoneuronal centers, as well as the afferent fibres to the various secondary sensory nuclei. Some centers like the superior and inferior olivary complexes are surrounded by fibrillary capsules which also stand out sharply as non-stained structures against the background. The olivo-cochlear bundle which has attracted so much attention as a possible cholinergic system (Desmedt and Monaco, 1961; Osen and Roth, 1969), did not show in an un-ambiguous manner in our material. It is also disconcerting that the superior olivary complex turned out to be a strikingly pale structure within the brain stem.

The only fibre bundle that was clearly stained in our material was a system of fibres already described by Olivier et al (1970a) which lies dorsal to the substantia nigra and that appears to correspond to non-myelinated fibres emerging from this center and directed toward more rostral levels, the striatum. These fibres form part of the "comb system" and can be seen as dark bands interposed between the fibres of the internal capsule.

In order to account for the difference between the stainability of fibre tracts with the AThChE method as recommended by Lewis (1961) and the lack of the stainability as it happened in our experiments, ist should be borne in mind that the technical procedures were different. In the material used for the present communication no fixation in formaldehyde was carried out. Since those authors who have described stained fibre bundles (Shute and Lewis, 1963a, 1963b, 1965, 1967; Lewis and Shute, 1967; Lewis et al., 1967; Krnjevic and Phillis, 1963; Krnjevic and Silver, 1963a, 1963b, 1965, 1966) appear to have fixed their material in formaldehyde, there is a possibility that the AThChE present in nerve fibres should require some kind of activation by formaldehyde in order to give a positive reaction (Taxi, 1952). One could also invoke some technical error on our part during the staining procedure. But, if this was the case, one would have to accept the fact that different patterns of stain distribution can be obtained depending on the type of technique used even when using the same substrate. An imperfect procedure could lead to the staining of either pseudo-cholinesterases or other substances capable of precipitating a copper salt during the incubation. But the selective non-stainability of any structure, *when others are stained*, must be regarded as significant whether the procedural error lies in not using formaldehyde or in any other step.

The Demarcation of Neuronal Groups. Even if it is difficult, at this stage, to interpret the biochemical and cytological significance of a positive AThChE stain, this histochemical technique constitutes, nevertheless, a valuable tool for the parcellation of the brain stem. In a previous communication (Ramon-Moliner and Nauta, 1966), it was stated that "a nucleus or center can be identified on the basis of any one of a variety of distinctive properties: specific functional effects following stimulation or lesion; histochemical properties; pigment content; specific afferent, efferent relationships; or, simply, evident cytological individuality." The above definition was put forward in an attempt to conceptualize and validate the notion of the reticular formation. At the time, it was pointed out that here is a vast region in the brain stem made out of subregions to which non of the requirements above listed appear to apply, and that, therefore a unitary notion appeared justified. This approach did not entail however, the possibility that, in the light of present and future evidence, the reticular formation should not eventually become parcellated into a number of territories with different hodological, physiological and histochemical properties.

The present work has shown that, particularly in the pontomesencephalic reticular formation, or tegmentum, the varying histochemical properties can provide a degree of parcellation which could not be suspected on the basis of previous evidence. For certain enzymes this histochemical variegation appears to reflect, in part, the uneven concentrations of nerve cells and fibres. Thus, in material stained for a demonstration of succinic dehydrogenase, Friede (1961) has produced evidence that this enzyme concentrates mostly in neuronal territories and that the regions rich in passing fibres are practically devoid of enzyme. This is not the case in AThChE material which shows (a) that compact neuronal centers can be either pale or intensely stained and (b) that the diffuse neuronal territories rich in passing fibres can also be intensely stained.

One of the arbitrary criteria that was used at one time to define the reticular formation was the fact that it is an admixture of neurons and passing fibres. Therefore, its "diffuse" characteristics would be of little significance since they could be the reflection of a varying degree of "neuronal dilution". In other words, a given cell group could still constitute a well-defined entity in spite of having a diffuse appearance due to the presence of such passing fibres. But the study of AThChE material demonstrates that "gradients" rather than sharp borderlines can be present, regardless of the presence or absence of such passing fibres. It also reveals that many centers which are well outlined in Golgi material, display equally sharp histochemical borderlines. This is not devoid of theoretical interest as it points, once again, towards the presence of two main categories of neuronal territories, open and closed (Mannen, 1960).

It can be said that the majority of the centers that form part of the isodendritic pool (Ramon-Moliner and Nauta, 1966) retain their diffuse borderlines in AThChE material, regardless of being positively or weakly stained. There are extremely well segregated allo-, or idiodentritic centers with equally sharp borderlines in AThChE material: the superior and inferior olivary complexes, the pontine nuclei, the nucleus interpeduncularis and the inferior colliculus. Other territories are not so well outlined but, nevertheless, can be individualized on dendroarchitectonic grounds. Often, they also stand out in AThChE material either as positively or weakly stained regions against a matrix within which they are, so to speak, encased. On the basis of its appearance in Golgi stained material, this matrix or core, was interpreted (Ramon-Moliner and Nauta, 1966) as a pool of pluripotential neurons which in the course of evolution remained diffusely distributed throught the brain stem, retaining generalized morphological features. The usually more circumscribed allodendritic and idiodendritic cell groups may have become segregated from this isodendritic pool as a result of being monopolized by specific connexions of functions.

In the medulla oblongata and the lower pons the diffuseness of the reticular or isodendritic core is not complicated by any outstanding variations in AThChE stainability. In the upper pons and the mesencephalon, this core displays both intensely and weakly stained areas. But these areas are seen blending with each other, as one could have expected by taking into account the considerable degree of overlapping of their dendritic fields. For this reason, we feel that the term "tegmentum" remains useful. It can still be subdivided into several regions which, in turn, can be coined on topographical grounds. But, on the other hand, it still conveys the idea of a *continuum* within which other better outlined centers of "nuclei" are embedded.

The fact that the various regions of the brain stem are so differently stained in AThChE material is not easy to correlate with any known functional or physiological differences. It has already been pointed out that all the motoneuronal centers and the majority of the secondary sensory centers are intensely stained. If the presence of AThChE reflects the presence, in vivo, of AChE involved in nervous conduction, these centers must be regarded as cholinoceptive, although not necessarily cholinergic. However, the possibility cannot be excluded that they could also be targets of several types of transmitters which could include ACh, as well as catecholamines and others. At present, in view of the many existing contradictions pointed out at the beginning of this discussion, it appears premature to attempt to correlate AThChE stainability and function.

Summary

A review of the acetylthiocholinesterase (AThChE) distribution in the brain stem of the cat was carried out on material stained with Koelle and Friedenwald's technique (1949) and with the cresylecht violet and luxol fast blue methods. The regional differences were outstanding and, in general, difficult to correlate with any existing hodological classifications. The only generalization that appears plausible applies to the motoneuronal centers which always showed a marked stain. The nuclei implicated in the auditory pathway were, with a few exceptions, poorer in enzyme than most other regions of the brain stem. The reticular formation (isodendritic core) retained its diffuse characteristics. In its caudal portion, no particular subdivisions could be proposed on the basis of the enzyme distribution. But, the rostral portion (tegmentum) could be subdivided into a number of sub-regions, according to their enzyme content. Nevertheless, no sharp borderlines could be established. For this reason, the term "tegmentum" has been retained in this report. A new nomenclature, which takes into account both histochemical and topographical factors, has been proposed to describe the various regions of this rostral portion of the reticular formation.

Acknowledgement. The author wishes to thank M. J. Ferrari for his patient technical contribution. He is particularly indebted to Mme. D. Desrochers for her valuable editing advice and secretarial help.

Abbreviations

(Labels in capital letters have been used in a consistent manner to refer to specific structures, regardless of the illustration where they appear. Small letters refer to details which are explained in the legend to the corresponding illustration and no attempt has been made to use them in consistent manner.)

A	nucleus ambiguus	PR	nuclei pararaphales medullae oblongatae
BC	brachium conjunctivum		
BP	brachium pontis	PV	nucleus principalis nervi trigeminis
CI	nucleus tegmentosus centralis inferioris		
		PYR	tractus pyramidalis
CL	nucleus cuneatus lateralis	Q	nucleus supratrigeminalis
CM	nucleus cuneatus medialis	RFC	formatio reticularis, pars caudalis
CR	corpus restiformis	RFG	formatio reticularis, pars gigantocellularis
CS	nucleus tegmentosus centralis superioris		
		RFM	formatio reticularis, pars magnocellularis
CSO	nuclei olivares superiores		
CV	nucleus cochlearis ventralis	RFP	formatio reticularis, pars parvocellularis
GC	griseum centrale		
GR	nucleus gracilis	S	nucleus supraspinatus
ICO	colliculus inferioris	SCO	colliculus superioris
IP	nucleus interpeduncularis	SV	nucleus spinalis nervi trigemini
MG	nucleus geniculatus medialis	TGCU	tegmentum cuneiformis
MLF	fasciculus longitudinalis medialis	TGDM	tegmentum dorsomedialis mesencephalii
MST	nucleus masticatorius		
NFL	nucleus funiculii lateralis ("lateral reticular nucleus")	TGEB	tegmentum entobrachialis
		TGIC	tegmentum infracollicularis
NG	substantia nigra	TGLM	tegmentum lateralis mesencephalii
NIV	nucleus trochlearis	TGPAR	tegmentum pararubralis
NLL	nucleus lemnisci lateralis	TGPBC	tegmentum peribrachialis, pars caudalis
NRM	nucleus raphe medullae oblongatae		
NT	nucleus trapezoidalis (medialis)	TGPL	tegmentum paralemniscalis
NVI	nucleus abducens	TGRG	tegmentum retrogeniculatus
NVII	nucleus nervi facialis	TGSB	tegmentum suprabrachialis
NXII	nucleus hypoglossii	TGSP	tegmentum suprapontinus
OIL	nucleus olivaris inferioris, pars lateralis (dorsalis)	U	tegmentum retrogeniculatus, pars caudalis ("nucleus parabigeminalis")
OIM	nucleus olivaris inferioris, pars medialis		
		VL	nucleus vestibularis lateralis
OIP	nucleus olivaris inferioris, pars principalis	VM	nucleus vestibularis medialis
		X	area X (nucleus cuneatus lateralis ?)
PNT	nuclei pontis		
PO	nucleus prepositus hypoglossii	Z	nucleus paraolivaris superioris ("lateral trapezoid nucleus")
PP	nucleus papillioformis		

References

Abrahams, V. C.: Histochemical localization of cholinesterase in some brain stem regions of the cat. J. Physiol. (Lond.) **165**, 55 P (1963).

Abrahams, V. C., Koelle, G. B., Smart, P.: Histochemical demonstration of cholinesterase in hypothalamus of dog. J. Physiol. (Lond.) **139**, 137–144 (1957).

Altman, J., Das, G. P.: Postnatal changes in the concentration and distribution of cholinesterase in the cerebellar cortex of rats. Exp. Neurol. **28**, 11–34 (1970).

Aprison, M. H., Takahashi, R., Folkerth, T. L.: Biochemistry of the avian central nervous system. I. The 5-hydroxy tryptophan decarboxilase, monoamine oxidase, and cholinacetylase-acetyl-cholinesterase systems in several discrete areas of pigeon brain. J. Neurochem. **11**, 341–350 (1964).

Austin, L., Phillis, J. W.: The distribution of cerebellar cholinesterases in several species. J. Neurochem. **12**, 709–727 (1965).

Barnes, J. M., Denz, F. A.: Experiemntal demyelination with organophosphorous compounds. J. Path. Bact. **65**, 597–605 (1953).

Barrnett, R. J.: The fine structural localization of acetylcholinesterase at the myoneural junction. J. Cell Biol. **12**, 247–262 (1962).

Bennett, E. L., Diamond, M. C., Morimoto, H., Herbert, M.: Acetylcholinesterase activity and weight measures in fifteen brain areas from six lines of rats. J. Neurochem. **13**, 563–572 (1966).

Berman, A. L.: The brain stem of the cat. A cytoarchitectonic atlas with stereotaxic coordinates. Madison, Wisconsin: University of Wisconsin Press 1968.

Bernsohn, J., Possley, L.: Cholinesterase in human and ruminant nervous tissue. Proc. Soc. exp. Biol. (N. Y.) **95**, 672–674 (1957).

Bloom, F. E., Barrnett, R. J.: The fine structural localization of cholinesterases in nervous tissue. Ann. N. Y. Acad. Sci. **144**, 613–625 (1967).

Bonichon, A.: Acetylcholinesterase dans la cellule et la fibre nerveuse au cours du développement. Bibl. anat. (Basel) **2**, 62–72 (1961).

Brightman, M. W., Albers, R. W.: Species differences in the distribution of extraneural cholinesterases within the vertebrate central nervous system. J. Neurochem. **3**, 244–250 (1959).

Brodal, A.: The reticular formation of the brain stem. Edinburgh and London: Oliver and Boyd 1958.

Brodal, A., Pompeiano, O., Walberg, F.: The vestibular nuclei and their connections. Anatomy and functional correlations. Edinburgh and London: Oliver and Boyd 1962.

Brown, L. M.: A thiocholine method for locating cholinesterase activity by Electron Microscopy. Bibl. anat. (Basel) **2**, 21–33 (1961).

Bull, C., Lawes, M., Leonard, M.: A modification of the thiocholine method for the demonstration of cholinesterases. Stain Technol. **32**, 59–61 (1957).

Burgen, A. S. V., Chipman, L. M.: Cholinesterase and succininic dehydrogenase in the central nervous system of the dog. J. Physiol. (Lond.) **114**, 296–305 (1951).

Cavanagh, J. B., Holland, P.: Cholinesterase in the chicken nervous system. Nature (Lond.) **190**, 735–736 (1961).

Cavanagh, J. B., Thompson, R. H. S., Webster, G. R.: The localization of pseudocholinesterase activity in nervous tissue. Quart. J. exp. Physiol. **39**, 185–197 (1954).

Chacko, L. W., Cerf, J. A.: Histochemical localization of cholinesterase in the amphybian spinal cord and alterations following ventral root section. J. Anat. (Lond.) **94**, 74–81 (1960).

Cohen, M.: Concentration of choline acetylase in conducting tissue. Arch. Biochem. **60**, 284–296 (1956).

Cordeau, J. P., Moreau, A., Beaubien, A., Laurin, C.: EEG and behavioral changes following microinjections of acetylcholine and adrenaline in the brain stem of cats. Arch. ital. Biol. **101**, 30–47 (1963).

Crawford, J. M., Curtis, D. R., Voorhoeve, P. E., Wilson, V. J.: Acetylcholine sensitivity of cerebellar neurons in the cat. J. Physiol. (Lond.) **186**, 139–165 (1966).

Curtis, D. R., Crawford, J. M.: Acetylcholine sensitivity of cerebellar neurons. Nature (Lond.) **206**, 516–517 (1965).

Curtis, D. R., Davis, R.: The excitation of lateral geniculate neurons by quaternary ammonium. J. Physiol. (Lond.) 165, 62–82 (1963).

Curtis, D. R., Eccles, R. M.: The excitation of Renshaw cells by pharmacogical agents applied electrophoretically. J. Physiol. (Lond.) 141, 435–445 (1958).

David, J. P., Murayama, S., Machne, X., Uma, K. R.: Evidence supporting cholinergic transmission at the lateral geniculate body of the cat. Int. J. Neuropharmacol. 2, 113–125 (1963).

De Robertis, E., Pellegrino de Iraldi, A., Rodriguez de Lores Arnaiz, G., Salganicoff, L.: Cholinergic and non-cholinergic nerve endings in the rat brain. Isolation and subcellular distribution of acetylcholine and acetylcholinesterase. J. Neurochem. 9, 23–25 (1962).

Desmedt, J. E., La Grutta, G.: The effect of selective inhibition of pseudocholinesterase on the spontaneous and evoked activity of the cat's cerebral cortex. J. Physiol. (Lond.) 136, 20–40 (1957).

Desmedt, J. E., Monaco, P.: Mode of action of the efferent olivocochlear bundle on the inner ear. Nature (Lond.) 192, 1263–1265 (1961).

Eccles, J. C., Eccles, R. M., Fatt, P.: Pharmacological investigations on a central synapse operated by acetylcholine. J. Physiol. (Lond.) 131, 154–169 (1956).

Eccles, J. C., Fatt, P., Koketsu, K.: Cholinergic and inhibitory synapses in a pathway from motor axon collaterals to motoneurons. J. Physiol. (Lond.) 126, 524–562 (1954).

Endröczi, E., Hartmann, G., Lissak, K.: Maturation of the acetylcholinesterase system of the brain stem in the newborn rat. Acta physiol. Acad. Sci. hung. 32, 307–315 (1967).

Eränkö, O., Rechardt, L., Hänninen, L.: Electron microscopic demonstration of cholinesterases in nervous tissue. Histochemie 8, 369–376 (1967).

Erulkar, S. D., Nichols, C. W., Popp, M. B., Koelle, G. B.: Renshaw elements: localization and acetylcholinesterase content. J. Histochem. Cytochem. 16, 128–135 (1968).

Essick, C. R.: The corpus pontobulbare — a hitherto undescribed nuclear mass in the human hindbrain. Amer. J. Anat. 7, 119–135 (1907).

Fahn, S., Côté, L. J.: Regional distribution of cholineacetylase in the brain of the rhesus monkey. Brain Res. 7, 323–325 (1968).

Feldberg, W.: Present views on the mode of action of acetylcholine in the central nervous system. Physiol. Rev. 25, 596–642 (1950).

Feldberg, W., Mann, T.: Properties and distribution of the enzyme system which synthesizes acetylcholine in nervous tissue. J. Physiol. (Lond.) 104, 411–425 (1946).

Feldberg, W., Vogt, M.: Acetylcholine synthesis in different regions of the central nervous system. J. Physiol. (Lond.) 107, 372–381 (1948).

Foldes, F. F., Zsigmond, E. K., Foldes, V. M., Erdös, E. G.: The distribution of acetylcholinesterase in the human brain. J. Neurochem. 9, 559–572 (1962).

Friede, R. L.: A histochemical atlas of tissue Oxidation in the brain stem of the cat. Basel and New York: Karger 1961.

Friede, R. L.: Topographic brain chemistry. New York: Academic Press 1966.

Friede, R. L.: A comparative histochemical mapping of the distribution of butyryl cholinesterase in the brain of four species of mammals, including man. Acta anat. (Basel) 66, 161–177 (1967).

Friede, R. L., Fleming, L. M.: A comparison of cholinesterase distribution in the cerebellum of several species. J. Neurochem. 11, 1–7 (1964).

Fukuda, T., Koelle, G. B.: The cytological localization of intracellular neuronal acetylcholinesterase. J. biophys. biochem. Cytol. 5, 433–440 (1959).

Geiger, R. S., Stone, W. G.: Localization of cholinesterases in adult mammalian cell cultures. Intern. J. Neuropharmacol. 1, 295–302 (1962).

George, R., Haslett, W. L., Jenden, D. J.: A cholinergic mechanism in the brain stem reticular formation: induction of paradoxical sleep. Intern. J. Neuropharmacol. 3, 541–552 (1964).

Gerebtzoff, M. A.: Cholinesterases. London: Pergamon Press 1959.

Giacobini, E.: The distribution and localization of cholinesterase in nerve cells. Acta physiol. scand. 45, Suppl. 156 (45 pp) (1959).

Girgis, M.: Distribution of cholinesterase in the basal rhinencephalic structures of the coypu. J. comp. Neurol. 129, 85–95 (1967).

Girgis, M.: Distribution of cholinesterase in the basal rhinencephalic structures of the grivet monkey. Acta anat. (Basel) **70**, 568–576 (1968).

Girgis, M.: Distribution of cholinesterase in the basal rhinencephalic structures of the Senegal bush baby. Acta anat. (Basel) **72**, 94–100 (1969).

Gomori, G.: Histochemical differentiation between sterases. Proc. Soc. exp. Biol. (N. Y.) **67**, 406 (1948a).

Gomori, G.: Histochemical demonstration of sites of cholinesterase activity. Proc. Soc. exp. Biol. (N. Y.) **68**, 354–358 (1948b).

Gomori, G.: Microscopic histochemistry. Chicago: Chicago University Press 1952.

Gomori, G., Chessick, R. D.: Esterases and phosphatases of the brain. A histochemical study. J. Neuropath. exp. Neurol. **12**, 387–396 (1953).

Gwyn, D. G., Wolstercroft, J. H.: Cholinesterase in the area subpostrema. A region adjacent to the area postrema in the cat. J. comp. Neurol. **133**, 289–308 (1968).

Hall, E., Geneser-Jensen, F. A.: Distribution of Acetylcholinesterase and monoamine oxidase in the amygdala of the guinea pig. Z. Zellforsch. **120**, 204–221 (1971).

Hard, W., Peterson, A. C.: The distribution of cholinesterase in nerve tissue of the dog. Anat. Rec. **108**, 57–70 (1950).

Harkmark, W.: The rhombic lip and its derivatives in relation to the theory of neurobiotaxis. In: Aspects of cerebellar anatomy (A. Brodal and J. Jansen, eds.), p. 264–284. Oslo: Grundt Tanum 1954).

Heading, C. E.: Cholinesterases and cholineacetylase in the nervous system of the rat. Brit. J. Pharmacol. **37**, 553P–554P (1969).

Hebb, C. O.: Cholineacetylase in mammalian and avian sensory systems. Quart. J. exp. Physiol. **40**, 176–186 (1955).

Hebb, C. O.: Cholinergic neurons in vertebrates. Nature (Lond.) **192**, 527–529 (1961).

Hebb, C. O., Silver, A.: Choline acetylase in the central nervous system of man and some animals. J. Physiol. (Lond.) **134**, 718–728 (1956).

Hebb, C. O., Waites, G. M.: Choline acetylase in antero and retrograde degeneration of a cholinergic neuron. J. Physiol. (Lond.) **132**, 667–671 (1956).

Hebb, C. O., Whittaker, V. P.: Intracellular distributions of acetylcholine and choline acetylase. J. Physiol. (Lond.) **142**, 187–196 (1958).

Hess, A.: The effects of eye removal on the development of cholinesterase in the inferior colliculus. J. exp. Zool. **144**, 11–19 (1960).

Hokin, L. E., Hokin, M. R.: Metabolism of phospholipids in vitro. Canad. J. Biochem. **34**, 349–360 (1956).

Holmes, R. L., Wolstencroft, J. H.: Cholinesterase in the medulla and pons of the cat. J. Physiol. (Lond.) **175**, 55P–56P (1964).

Holmstedt, B.: A modification of the thiocholine method for the determination of cholinesterase. Acta physiol. scand. **40**, 322–337 (1957).

Hyyppä, M.: Histochemically demonstrable esterase activity in the hypothalamus of the developing rat. Histochemie **20**, 29–39 (1969).

Iijima, K., Bourne, G. H.: Histochemical studies of esterases, monoaminoxidase, and dephosphorilating enzymes in the area postrema of squirrel monkey. Acta histochem. (Jena) **29**, 349–363 (1968).

Iijima, K., Shanta, T. R., Bourne, G. H.: Histochemical studies of the pigments and distribution of various enzymes in the dorsal vagal nucleus and hypoglossal nucleus of squirrel monkey. Acta histochem. (Jena) **32**, 18–36 (1969).

Kasa, P., Joo, F., Csillik, B.: Histochemical localization of acetylcholinesterase in the cat cerebellar cortex. J. Neurochem. **12**, 31–37 (1965).

King, E. J., Sperri, W. M.: Biochemistry Handbook. London: Spon 1961.

Koelle, G. B.: The histochemical differentiation of types of cholinesterase and their localization in the tissue of the cat. J. Pharmacol. exp. Ther. **100**, 158–179 (1950).

Koelle, G. B.: The elimination of enzymatic diffusion artefacts in the histochemical localization of cholinesterases and a survey of their cellular distribution. J. Pharmacol. exp. Ther. **103**, 153–171 (1951).

Koelle, G. B.: Histochemical localization of cholinesterases in the central nervous system of the rat. J. Pharmacol. exp. Ther. **106**, 401 (1952).

Koelle, G. B.: The histochemical cemonstration of acetylcholinesterase in cholinergic, adre-
nercig and sensory neurons. J. Pharmacol. exp. Ther. 114, 167–184 (1955).

Koelle, G. B., Davis, R., Gromadzki, C. G.: Electron microscopic localization of cholinesterase
by means of gold salts. Ann. N. Y. Acad. Sci. 144, 613–625 (1967).

Koelle, G. B., Friedenwald, J. S.: A method for localizing cholinesterase activity. Proc. Soc.
exp. Biol. (N. Y.) 70, 617–622 (1949).

Koelle, G. B., Gromadzki, C. G.: Comparison of the gold thiocholine and thioloacetic acid
methods for the histochemical localization of acetylcholinesterase and cholinesterases.
J. Histochem. Cytochem. 14, 443–454 (1966).

Krnjevic, K.: Cholinesterase staining in the cerebral cortex. J. Physiol. (Lond.) 165, 3P–4P
(1963b).

Krnjevic, K.: A histochemical study of cholinergic fibres in the cerebral cortex. J. Anat.
(Lond.) 99, 711–759 (1965).

Krnjevic, K.: Acetylcholinesterase in the developing forebrain. J. Anat. (Lond.) 100, 63–89
(1966).

Krnjevic, K., Phillis, J. W.: Acetylcholine sensitive cells in the cerebral cortex. J. Physiol.
(Lond.) 166, 296–327 (1963).

Krnjevic, K., Silver, A.: The distribution of "cholinergic" fibres in the cerebral cortex. J.
Physiol. (Lond.) 168, 39P–40P (1963a).

La Torre, J. C.: Effect of differential environmental enrichment on brain weight and on
acetylcholinesterase and cholinesterase activities in mice. Exp. Neurol. 22, 493–503 (1968).

Lehrer, G. M., Ornstein, L. A.: A diazo coupling method for electron microscopic localization
of cholinesterase. J. biophys. biochem. Cytol. 6, 399–406 (1959).

Lewis, P. R.: The effect of varying the conditions in the Koelle technique. Bibl. anat. (Basel)
2, 11–20 (1961).

Lewis, P. R.: The cholinergic limbic system: projection to hippocampal formation, medial
cortex, nuclei of the ascending reticular system, the subfornical organ, and supraoptic
crest. Brain 90, 521–540 (1967).

Lewis, P. R.: An electron microscopic study of cholinesterase distribution in the rat adrenal
medulla. J. Microscopy 89, 181–192 (1969).

Lewis, P. R., Flumerfelt, B. A.: The pseudocholinesterase containing neurons in the rat
hypoglossal nucleus. J. Anat. (Lond.) 106, 189 (1970).

Lewis, P. R., Scott, J. A., Navaratnam, V.: Localization in the dorsal motor nucleus of the
vagus in the rat. J. Anat. (Lond.) 107, 197–208 (1970).

Lewis, P. R., Shute, C. C. D.: The distribution of cholinesterase in cholinergic neurons demonstrated with the electron microscope. J. Cell Sci. 1, 381–390 (1966).

Lewis, P. R., Shute, C. C. D., Silver, A.: Confirmation from choline acetylase analysis of a
massive cholinergic innervation to the rat hippocampus. J. Physiol. (Lond.) 191, 215–224
(1967).

MacIntosh, F. C.: The distribution of acetylcholine in the peripheral and the central nervous
system. J. Physiol. (Lond.) 99, 436–442 (1941).

MacIntosh, F. C., Oborin, P. E.: Release of acetylcholine from intact cerebral cortex, p.
580–581. Abstr. XIX Intern. Physiol Congr. 1953.

Maletta, G. J., Timires, P. S.: Acetylcholinesterase activity in optic structures after complete
light deprivation from birth. Exp. Neurol. 19, 513–518 (1967).

Malmgren, H., Sylven, B.: On the chemistry of the thiocholine method of Koelle. J. Histochem. Cytochem. 3, 441–445 (1955).

Mannen, H.: Noyau fermé et noyau ouvert. Arch. ital. Biol. 98, 333–350 (1960).

Manolov, S.: Comparative investigations on cholinesterase activity in cranial and spinal
motoneurons. Acta histochem. (Jena) 32, 37–49 (1967).

Mathisen, J. S., Blackstad, T. W.: Cholinesterase in the hippocampal region. Acta anat.
(Basel) 56, 216–253 (19654).

McLennan, H.: The release of acetylcholine and of 3-hydroxytyramine from the caudate
nucleus. J. Physiol. (Lond.) 174, 152–161 (1964).

McLennan, H.: Cholinesterase in the feline red nucleus. J. Neuropharmacol. 8, 489–490 (1969).

Mehler, W. R.: Some neurological species differences. Ann. N. Y. Acad. Sci. 167, 424–468
(1969).

Miller, E., Reinwall, J., Brouwer, J., Earl, F. L., Curtis, J. M.: Regional distribution of cholinesterase in the central nervous system of miniature swine. Amer. J. vet. Res. **30**, 2037–2039 (1969).

Mitchell, J. F.: The spontaneous and evoked release of acetylcholinesterase from the cerebral cortex. J. Physiol. (Lond.) **165**, 98–116 (1963).

Morest, D. K.: A study of the area postrema with Golgi methods. Amer. J. Anat. **107**, 291–303 (1960).

Morest, D. K.: The collateral system of the medial nucleus of the trapezoid body of the cat; its neuronal architecture and relation to the olivocochlear bundle. Brain Res. **9**, 288–311 (1968).

Nachmansohn, D.: Actions on axons and evidence for the role of acetylcholine in axonal conduction. Chap. 15 in: Cholinesterases and anticholinesterase agents, Handbuch der experimentellen Pharmakologie Ergänzungswerk (G. B. Koelle). Berlin-Göttingen-Heidelberg: Springer 1964.

Nachmansohn, D.: Proteins in excitable membranes. Science **168**, 1059–1066 (1970).

Naïk, N. T.: Technical variations in Koelle's histochemical method for demonstrating cholinesterase activity. Quart. J. micr. Sci. **104**, 89–100 (1963).

Navaratnam, V., Lewis, P. R.: Cholinesterase containing neurons in the spinal cord of the rat. Brain Res. **18**, 411–425 (1970).

Okinaka, S., Yoshikawa, M., Uono, M., Muro, T., Mozai, T., Igata, A., Tanabe, H., Ueda, S., Tomonage, M.: Distribution of cholinesterase activity in the human cerebral cortex. Amer. J. Physiol. Med. **40**, 135–145 (1961).

Olivier, A., Parent, A,. Poirier, L. J.: Identification of the thalamic nuclei on the basis of their cholinesterase content in the monkey. J. Anat. (Lond.) **106**, 37–50 (1970b).

Olivier, A., Parent, A., Simard, H., Poirier, L. J.: Cholinesterasic striatopallidal and striatonigral efferents in the cat and the monkey. Brain Res. **18**, 273–282 (1970a).

Olszewski, J., Baxter, D.: Cytoarchitecture of the human brain stem. Basel and New York: S. Karger 1954.

Ord, M. G., Thompson, R. H. S.: Pseudocholinesterase activity in the central nervous system. J. Biochem. **51**, 245–251 (1952).

Osen, K. K., Roth, K.: Histochemical localization of cholinesterases in the cochlear nuclei of the cat, with notes on the origin of acetylcholinesterase positive afferents and the superior olive. Brain Res. **16**, 165–185 (1969).

Palmer, A. C., Ellerker, A. R.: Histochemical localization in the brain stem of sheep. Quart. J. exp. Physiol. **46**, 344–352 (1961).

Papp, M.: Acetylcholinesterase activity of the human lower brain stem with special reference to the reticular formation. Acta morph. Acad. Sci. hung. **16**, 375–390 (1968).

Papp, M., Bozsik, G.: Comparison of the cholinesterase activity of the lower brain stem of cat and rabbit. J. Neurochem. **13**, 697–703 (1966).

Pavin, H. A., Zacks, S. I., Seligman, A. M.: The histochemical localization of acetylcholinesterase in nervous tissue. J. Phamacol. exp. Ther. **107**, 37–53 (1953).

Pavin, R.: Cholinesterases in reticular cells. J. Neurochem. **12**, 515–518 (1965).

Peppler, W. J., Pearse, A. G. E.: The histochemistry of the esterases of rat brain with special reference to those of the hypothalamic nuclei. J. Neurochem. **1**, 193–202 (1956).

Pope, A.: Quantitative distribution of dipeptidase and acetylcholinesterase in architectonic layers of rat cerebral cortex. J. Neurophysiol. **15**, 115–129 (1952).

Quastel, J. H.: Acetylcholine distribution and synthesis in the central nervous system. In: K. A. C. Elliott, J. H. Page, and J. H. Quastel (eds.), Neurochemistry. Springfield, Ill.: Thomas 1962.

Ramon y Cajal, S.: Histologie du système nerveux. Paris: Maloine 1911.

Ramon-Moliner, E.: La différentiation morphologique des neurones. Arch. ital. Biol. **105**, 149–188 (1967).

Ramon-Moliner, E.: The morphology of dendrites. In: Structure and function of nervous tissue (G. H. Bourne, ed.), p. 205–267. New York: Academic Press 1968.

Ramon-Moliner, E.: The leptodendritic neuron: its distribution and significance. Ann. N. Y. Acad. Sci. **167**, 65–70 (1969).

Ramon-Moliner, E., Nauta, W. J. H.: The isodendritic core of the brain stem. J. comp. Neurol. **126**, 311–336 (1966).

Roessman, U., Friede, R. L.: Changes in butyryl cholinesterase activity in reactive glia. Neurology (Minneap.) **16**, 123–129 (1966).

Sawyer, C. H.: Cholinesterases in degenerating and regenerating peripheral nerves. Amer. J. Physiol. **146**, 246–253 (1946).

Sharma, N. N.: Studies on the histochemical distribution of simple esterase and cholinesterases in the olfactory bulb of the rat. Acta anat. (Basel) **69**, 168–175 (1968).

Shen, S., Greenfield, P., Boell, E.: The distribution of cholinesterase in the frog brain. J. comp. Neurol. **102**, 717–734 (1955).

Shen, S. C., Greenfield, P., Sippel, T.: Application of histochemical technic for cholinesterase to paraffin sections. Proc. Soc. exp. Biol. (N.Y.) **81**, 452–455 (1952).

Shute, C. C. D., Lewis, P. R.: The salivatory center in the rat. J. Anat. (Lond.) **94**, 59–73 (1960).

Shute, C. C. D., Lewis, P. R.: The use of cholinesterase techniques combined with operative procedures to follow nervous pathways in the brain. Bibl. anat. (Basel) **2**, 34–49 (1961).

Shute, C. C. D., Lewis, P. R.: Cholinesterase containing systems of the brain of the rat. Nature (Lond.) **199**, 1160–1164 (1963a).

Shute, C. C. D., Lewis, P. R.: The cholinergic corticopetal radiations of the forebrain. J. Anat. (Lond.) **97**, 476–477 (1963b).

Shute, C. C. D., Lewis, P. R.: Cholinesterase containing pathways of the hindbrain: afferent cerebellar and centrifugal cochlear fibres. Nature (Lond.) **205**, 242–247 (1965).

Shute, C. C. D., Lewis, P. R.: Electron microscopy of cholinergic terminals and acetylcholinesterase containing neurons in the hippocampal formation of the rat. Z. Zellforsch. **69**, 334–343 (1966).

Shute, C. C. D., Lewis, P. R.: The ascending cholinergic reticular system: neocortical, olfactory and subcortical projections. Brain **90**, 497–520 (1967).

Shute, C. C. D., Lewis, P. R.: Localization of cholinesterase in monkey brain. J. Anat. (Lond.) **104**, 186–187 (1969).

Silver, A.: Cholinesterases of the central nervous system with special reference to the cerebellum. Int. Rev. Neurobiol. **10**, 57–109 (1967).

Siou, G.: Distribution normale et variation expérimentale de l'activité cholinestérasique au niveau des tubercules quadrijumeaux antérieurs chez la souris. C. R. Acad. Sci. (Paris) **246**, 315–317 (1958).

Snell, R. S.: The histochemical localization of cholinesterase in the central nervous system. Bibl. anat. (Basel) **2**, 50–58 (1961).

Snider, R. S., Niemer, W. T.: A stereotaxic atlas of the cat brain. Chicago and London: Chicago University Press 1961.

Spector, W. S.: Handbook of biological data. Saunders, Pa. 1956.

Stolk, A.: Distribution of cholinesterase in the nervous system of Iguana iguana. Proc. kon. med. Akad. Wet. Amsterdam **65**, 186–198 (1962).

Taber, E.: The cytoarchitecture of the brain stem of the cat. J. comp. Neurol. **116**, 27–69 (1961).

Taber, E., Brodal, A., Walberg, F.: The raphe nuclei of the brain stem in the cat. J. comp. Neurol. **114**, 161–187 (1960).

Taxi, J.: Action du formol sur l'activité de diverses préparations de cholinestérase. J. Physiol. (Paris) **44**, 595–599 (1952).

Whittaker, M.: The serum cholinesterase variants. Differentiation by means of formaldehyde. Clin. chim. Acta **26**, 141–145 (1969).

Whittaker, V. P., Sheridan, M. N.: The morphology and acetylcholine content of isolated cerebral cortical synaptic vesicles. J. Neurochem. **12**, 363–372 (1965).

Winkler, C., Potter, A.: An anatomical guide to experimental researches on the cat's brain. Amsterdam Versluys 1914.

Wurzel, M.: The physiological role of cholinesterase at cholinergic receptor sites. Ann. N. Y. Acad. Sci. **144**, 694–704 (1967).

Zachs, S. I., Blumberg, J. M.: The histochemical localization of acetylcholinesterase in the fine structure of neuromuscular junctions of mouse and human intercostal muscle. J. Histochem. Cytochem. **9**, 317–324 (1961).

Subject Index